My daughter is teaching me how to use the internet. She told me to type any question into the Google search bar. 'I wrote Can I have a nice cup of tea, please?'

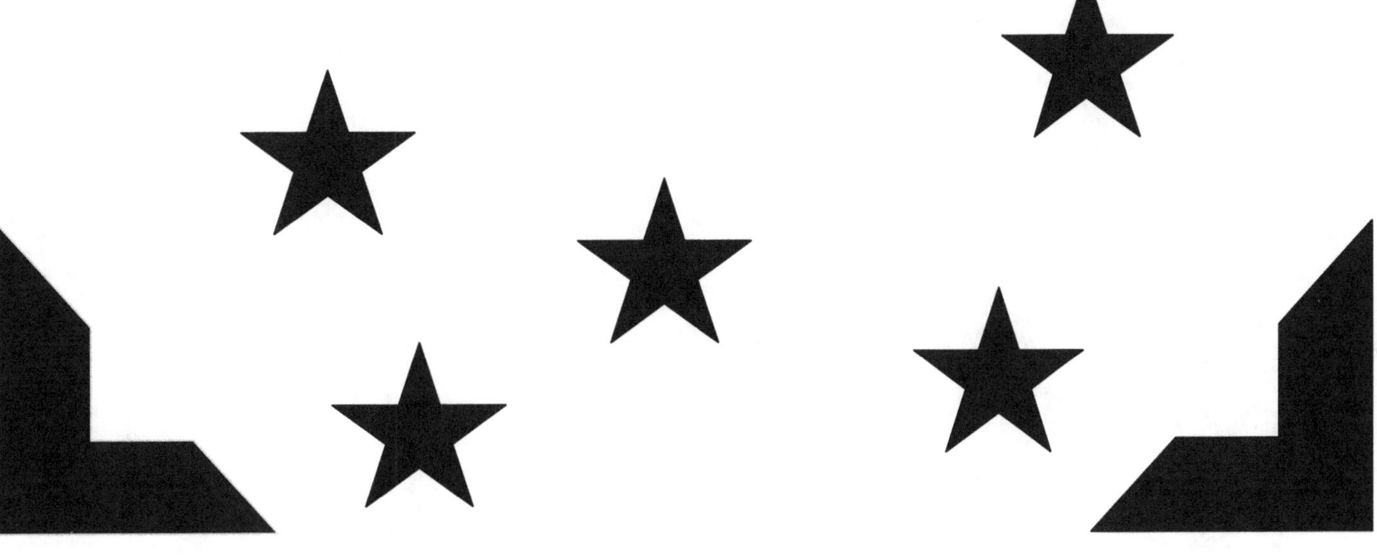

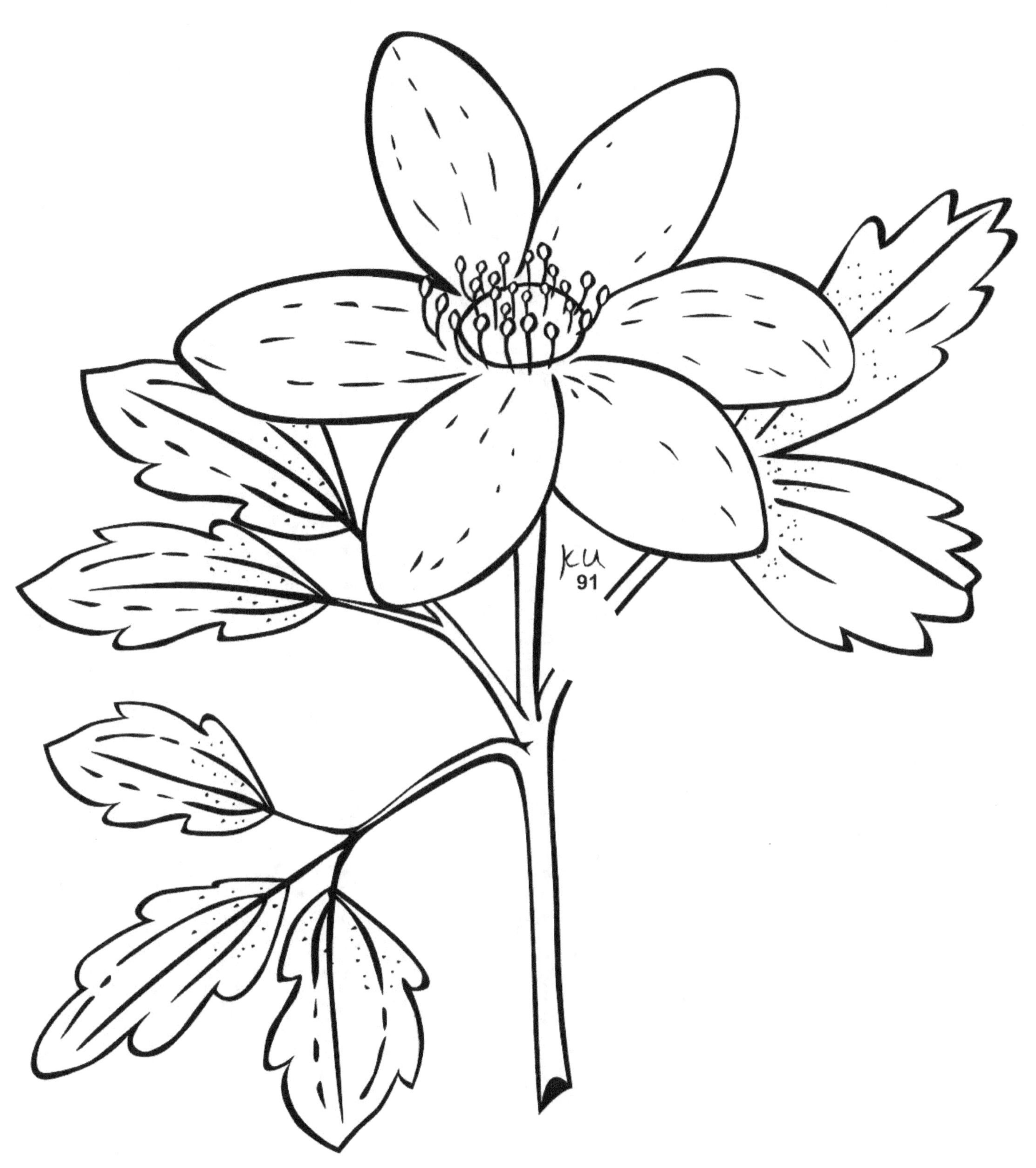

A teenager and her foreign grandmother were on their way to the supermarket.

Shall we cross here Grandma?

"Of course not dear, look what happened to the poor zebra."

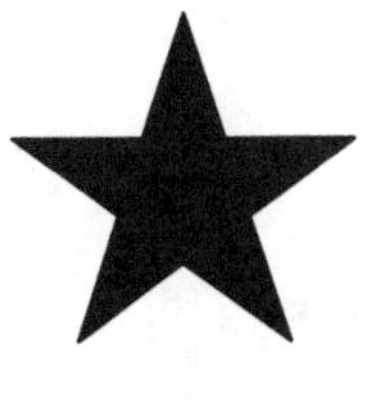

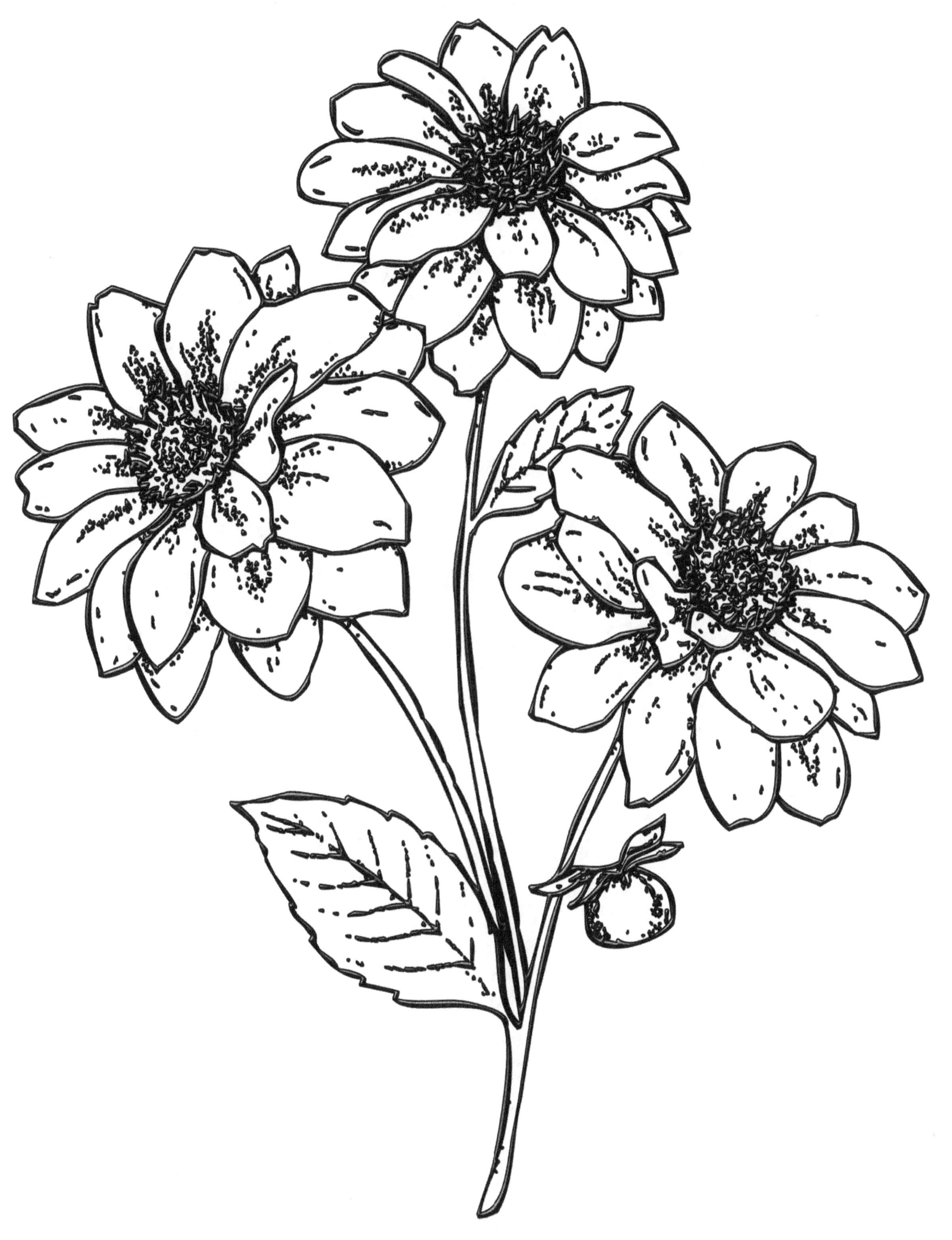

A grandmother asked her Grandson "Can you pass me my glasses, please?"
When the grandson gave his grandmother her glasses his Grandmother said " Thank you Jacob, you know you are such a great grandson much better than your brother Adam.

___________________________ _

"Put your glasses on Grandma, I am Adam."

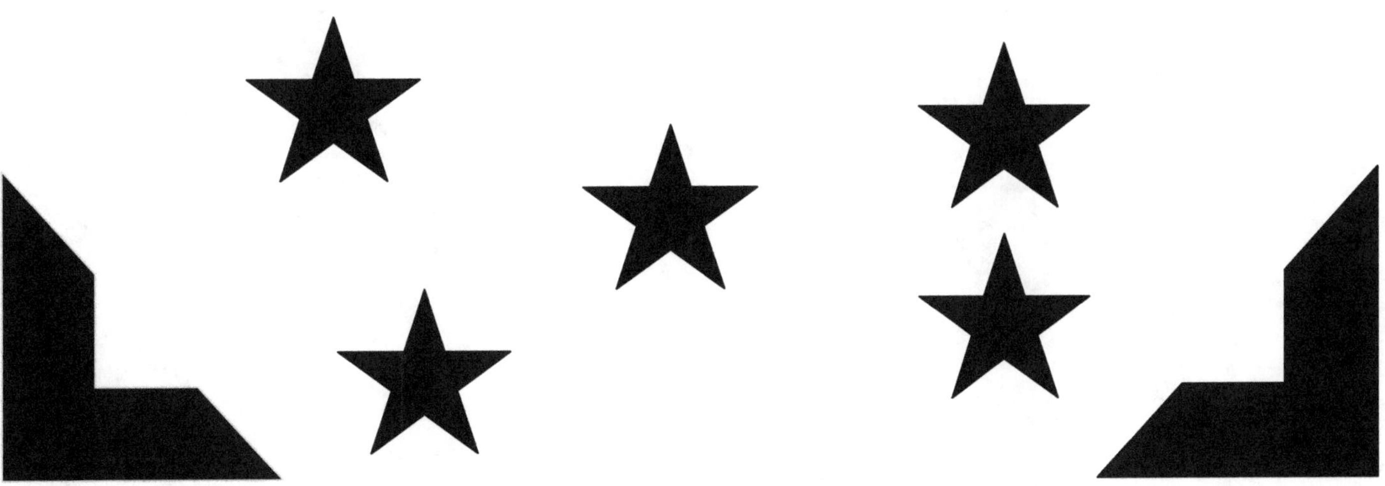

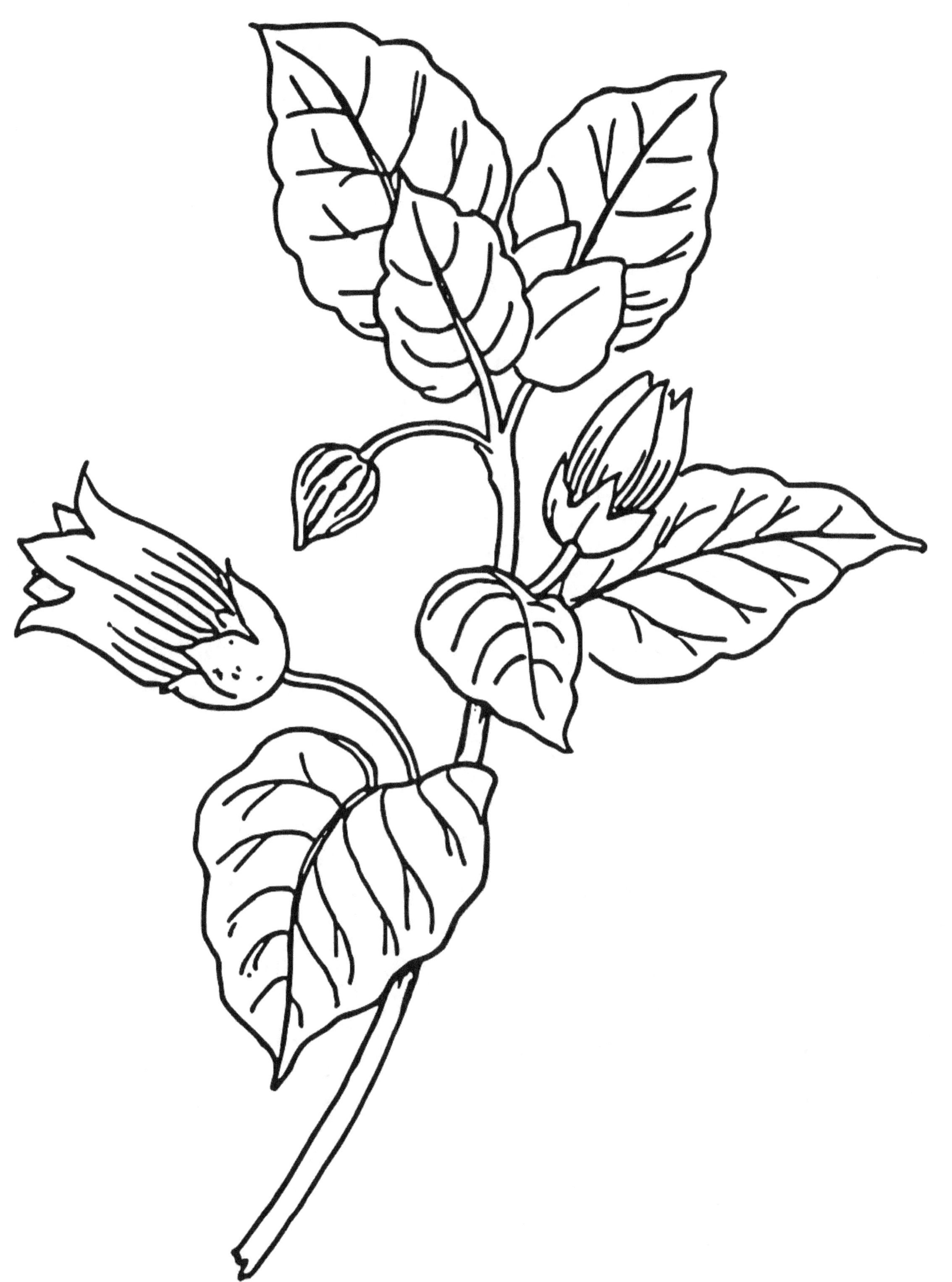

I am old enough to make my own decisions, just not young enough to remember what I decided.

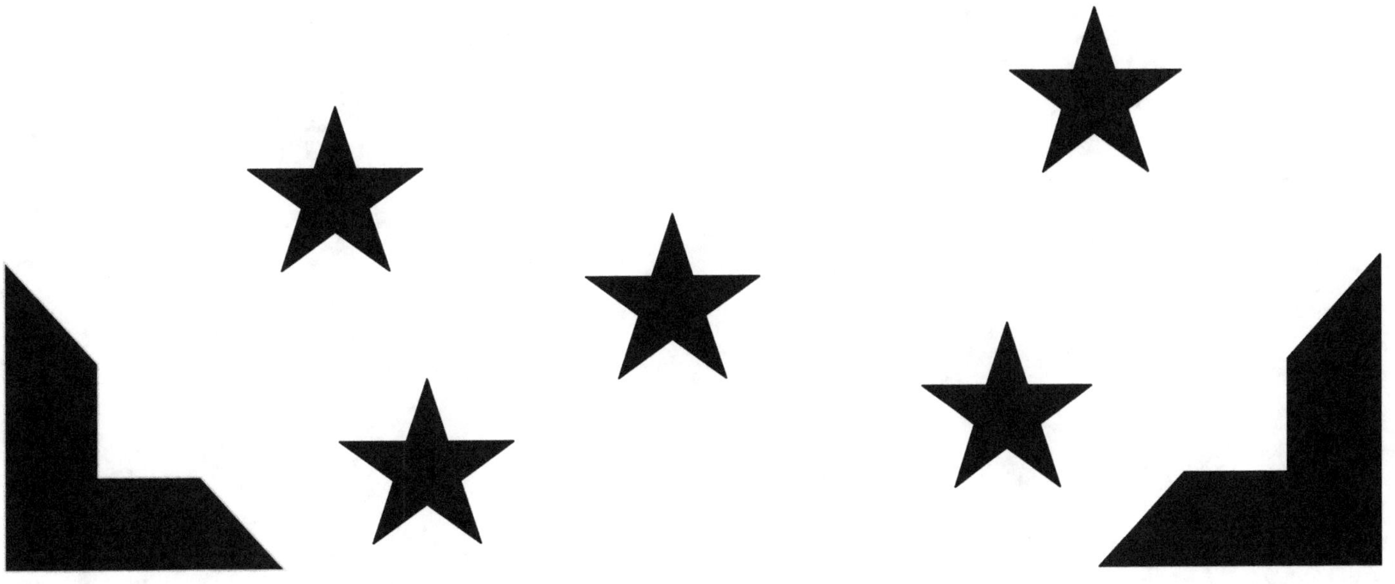

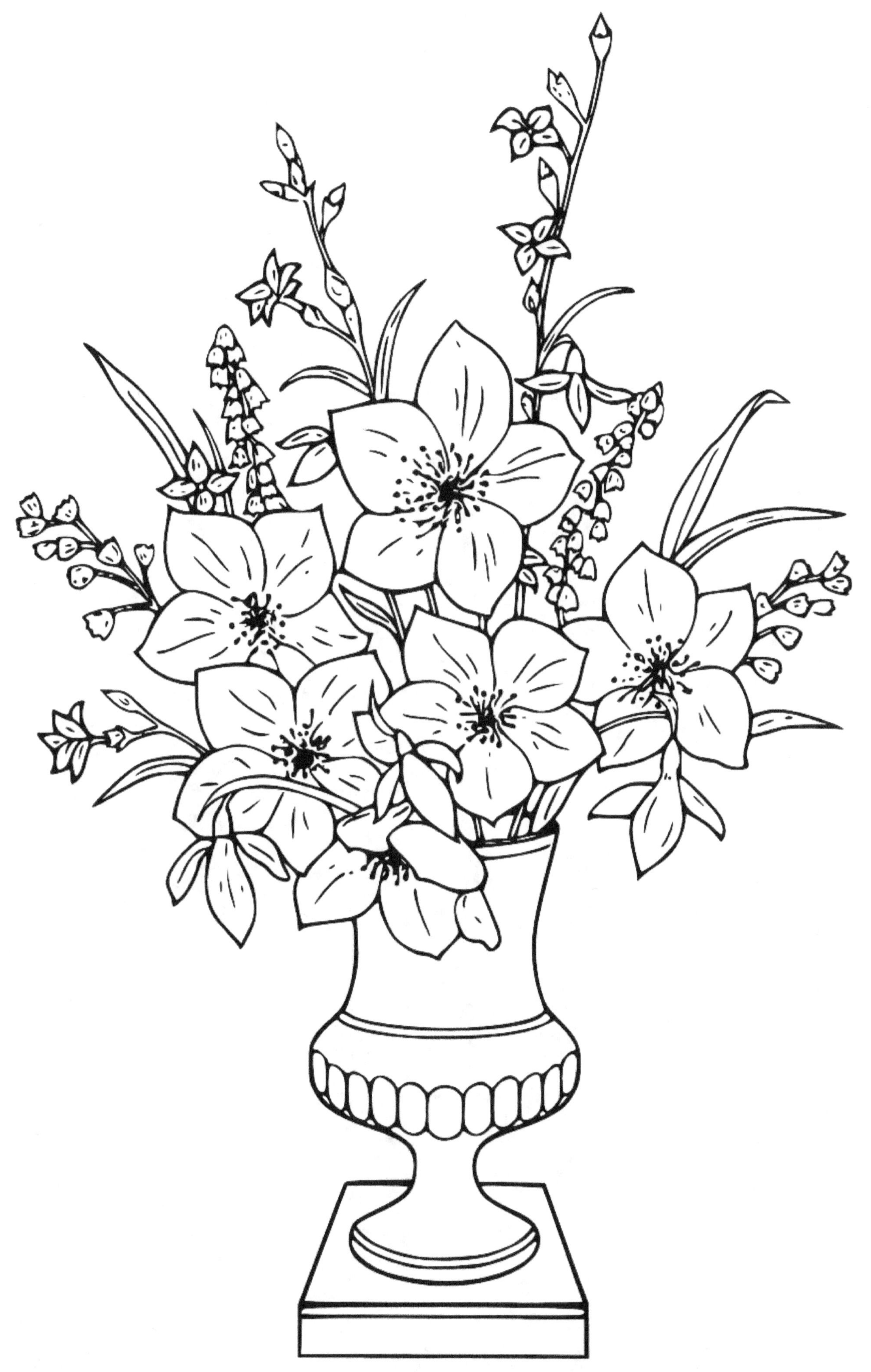

Grandma, Did you
hear about the new
movie constipation?

It hasn't come out
yet!

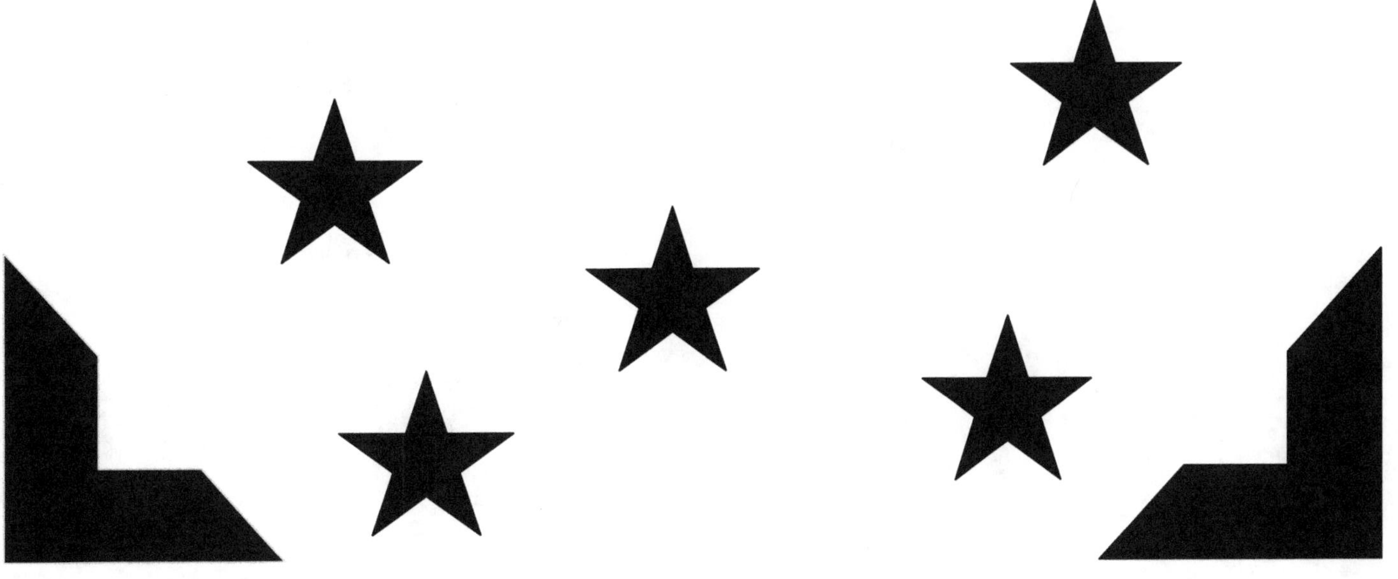

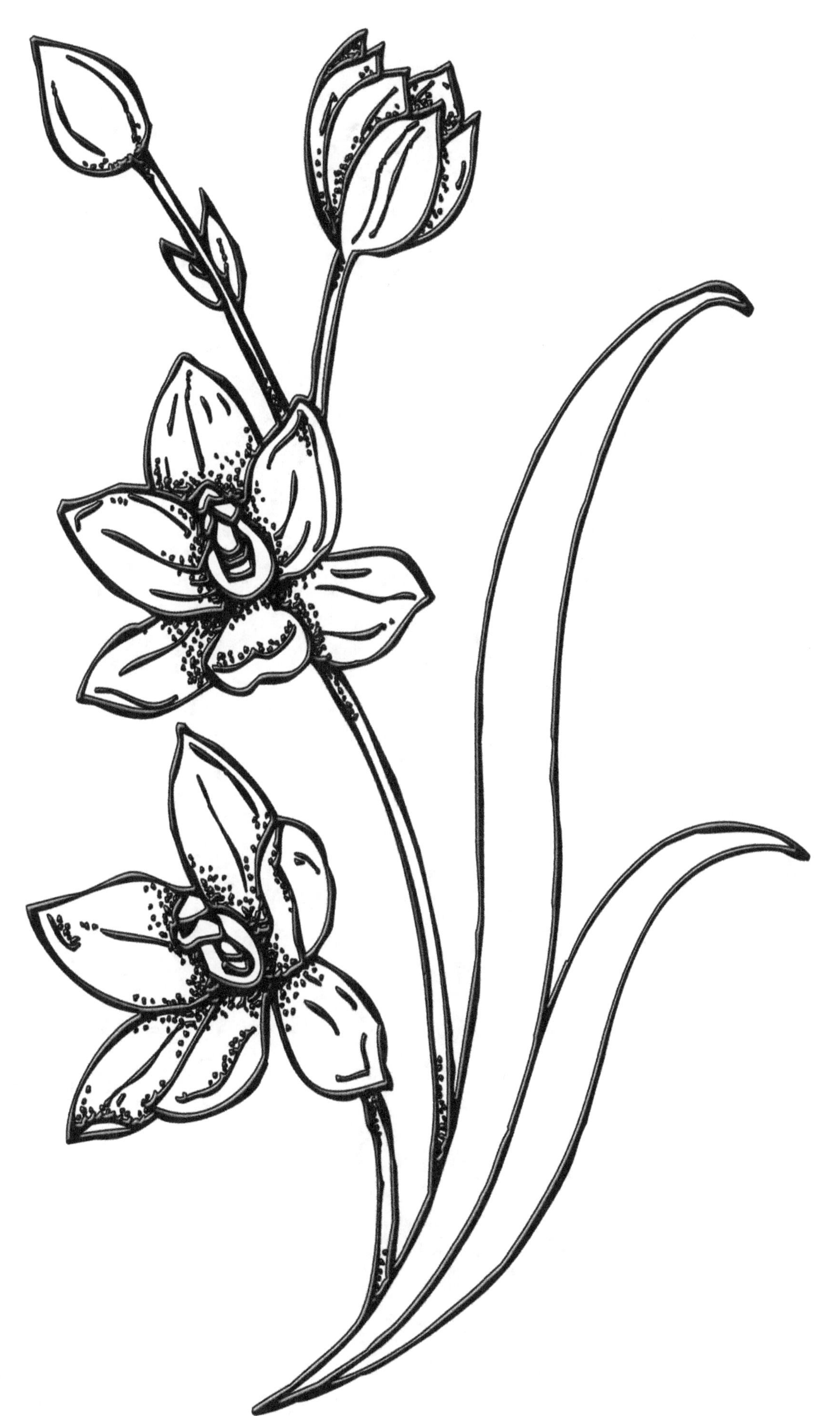

My doctor told me that I should lose some weight. So I have officially started the See Food Diet.

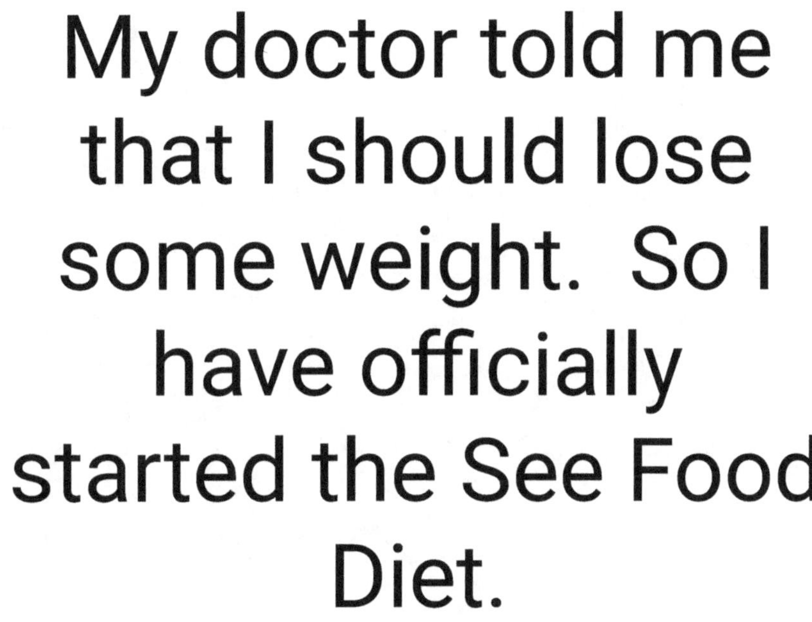

Any food I see, I eat!

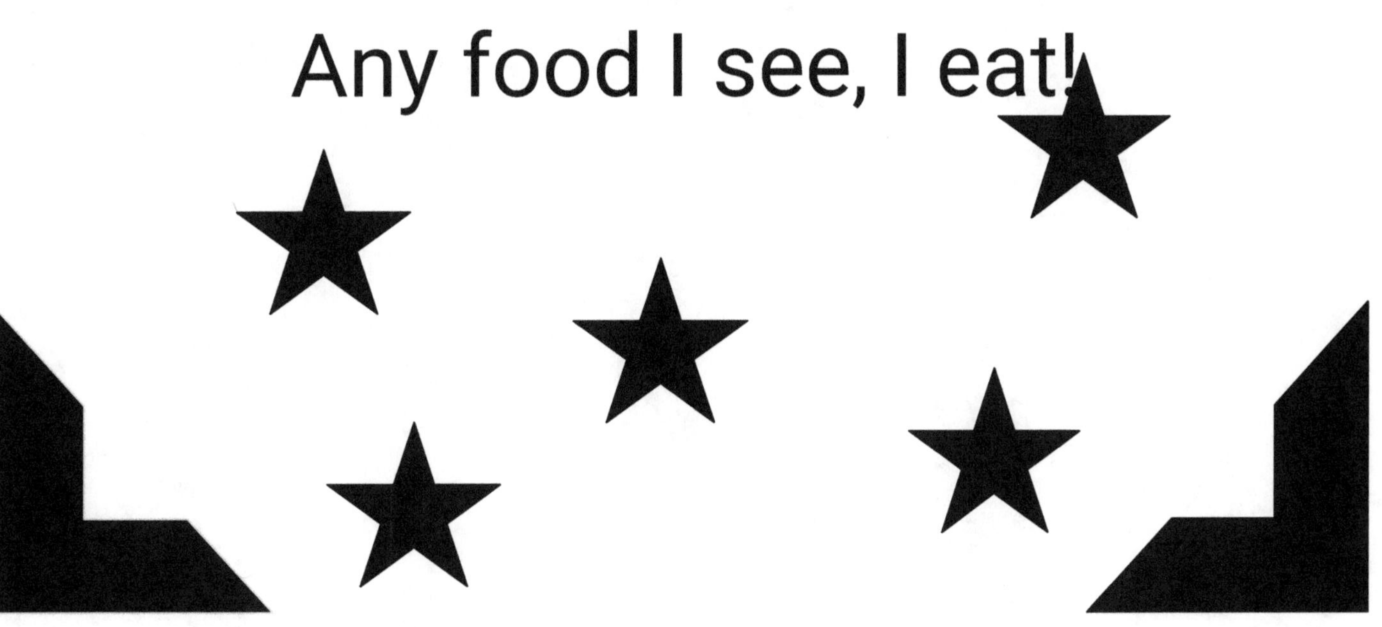

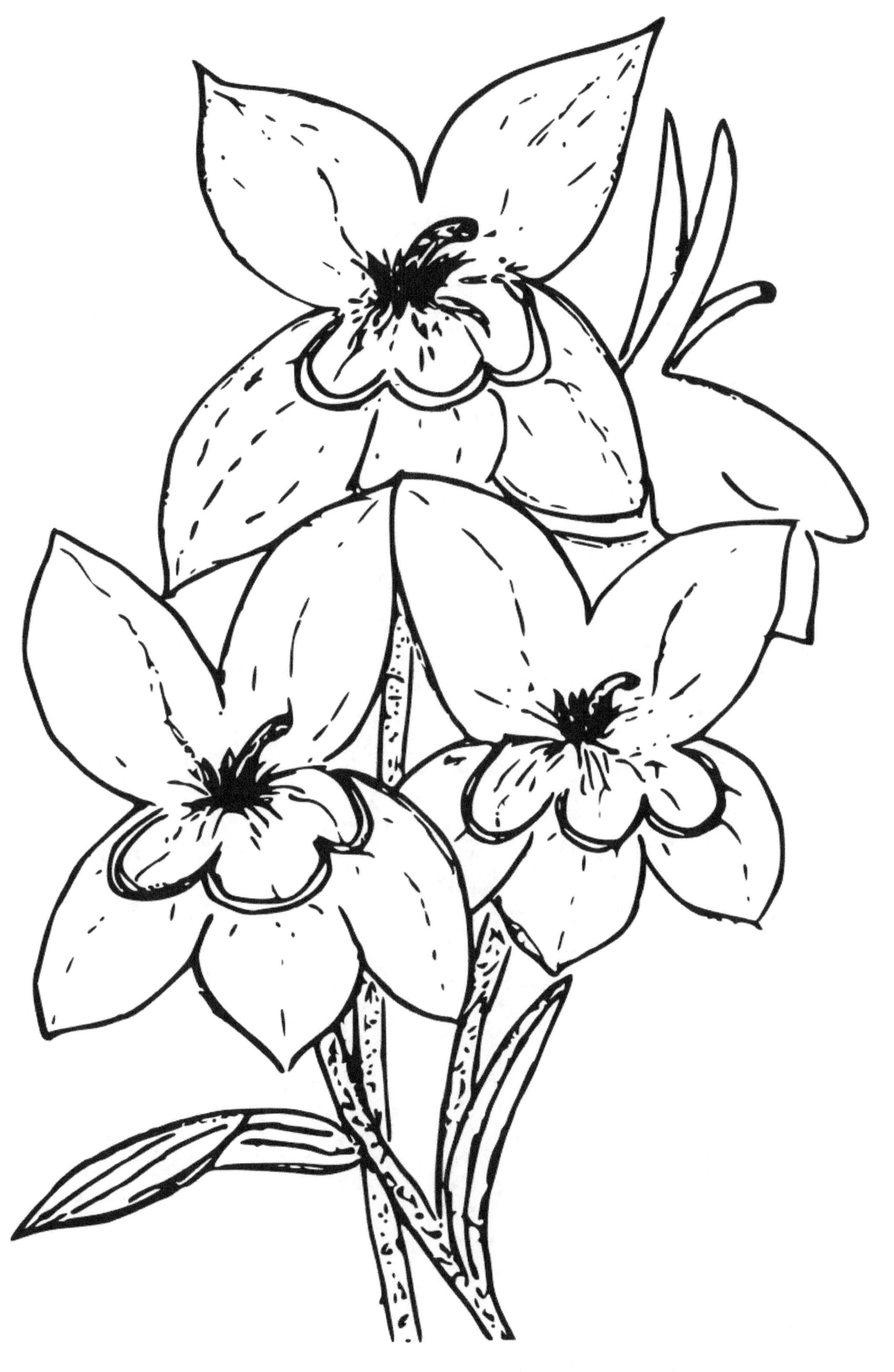

Whenever I can't
remember
someone's name I
just say things like
sugar, lovely, my
dear.

It works every time!

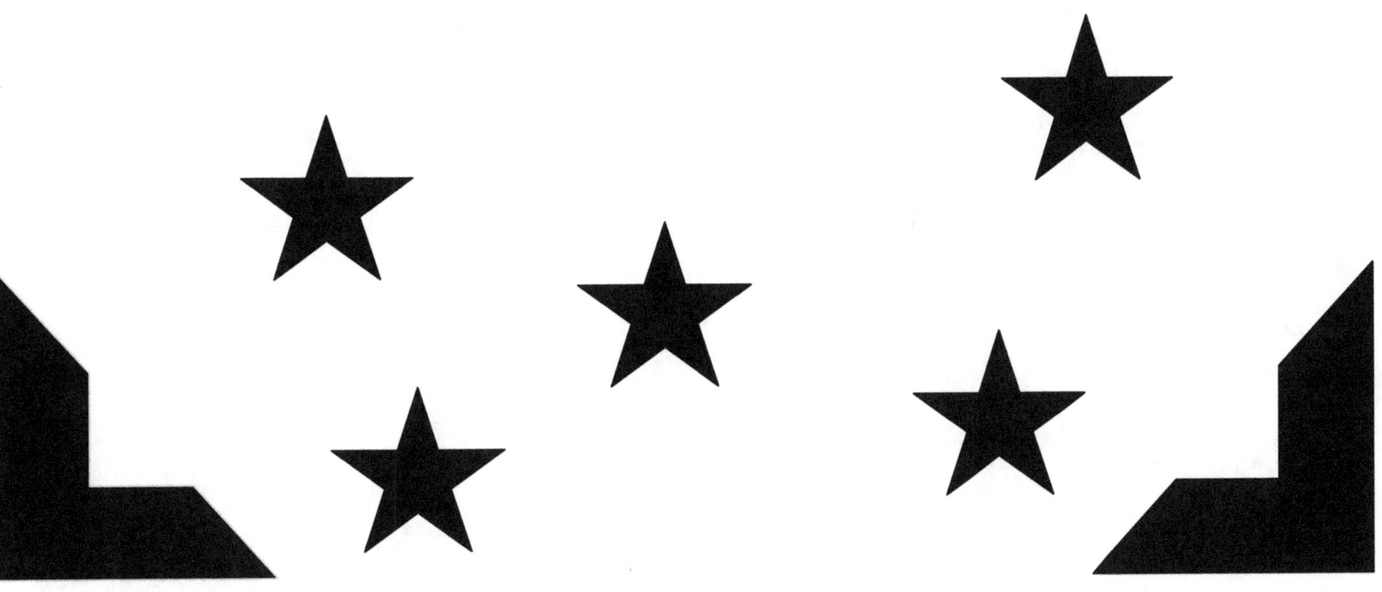

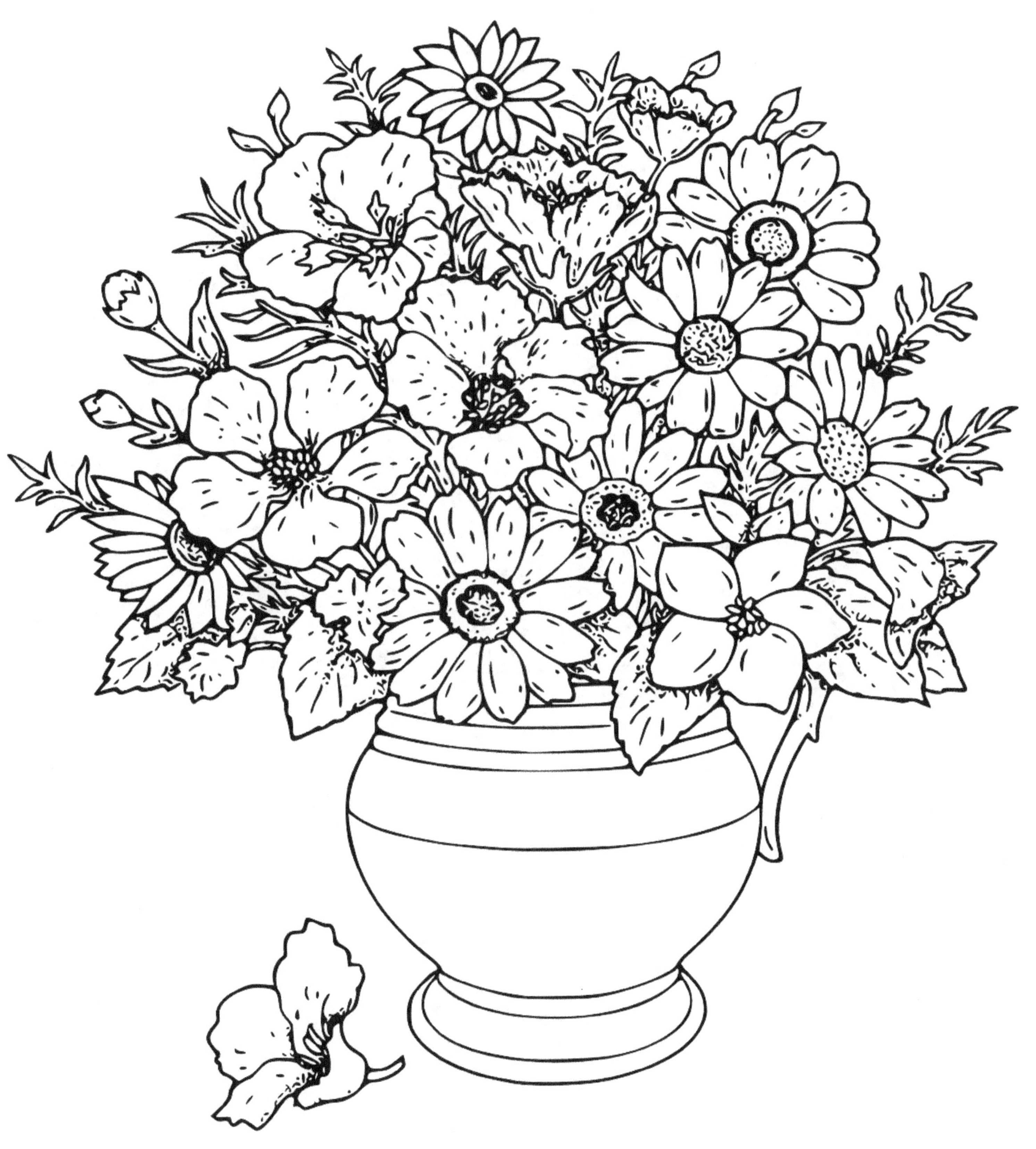

I do miss having a
good laugh.
Now I have to be
careful because I
don't want my teeth
to fall out!

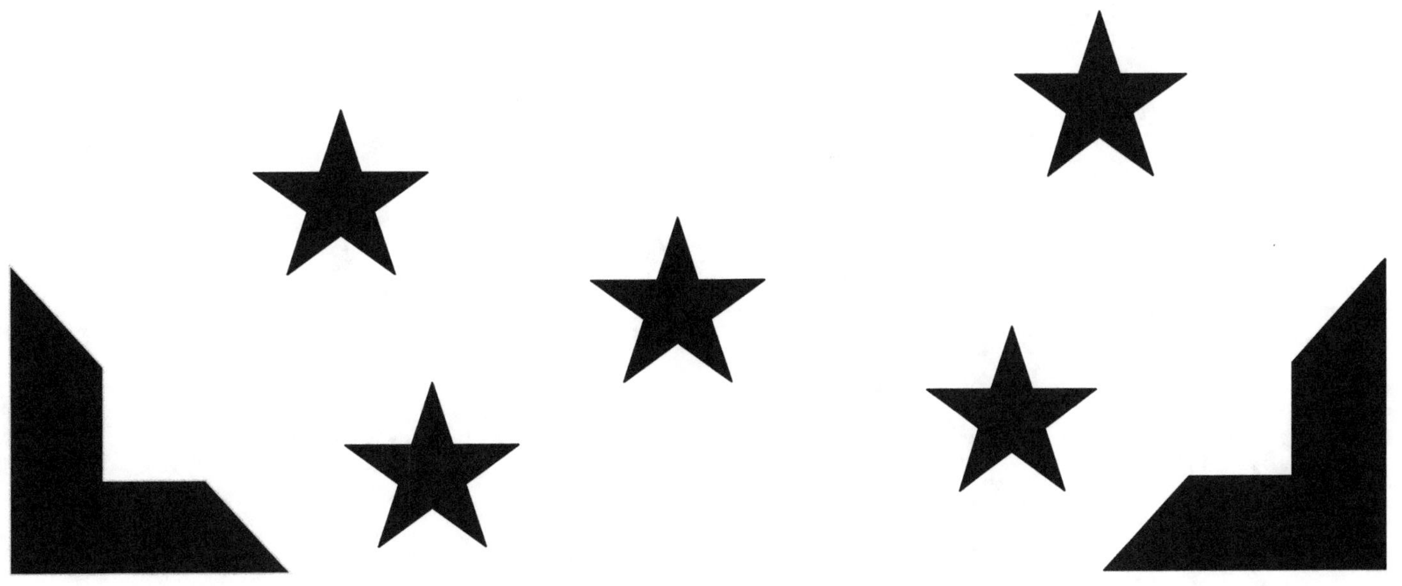

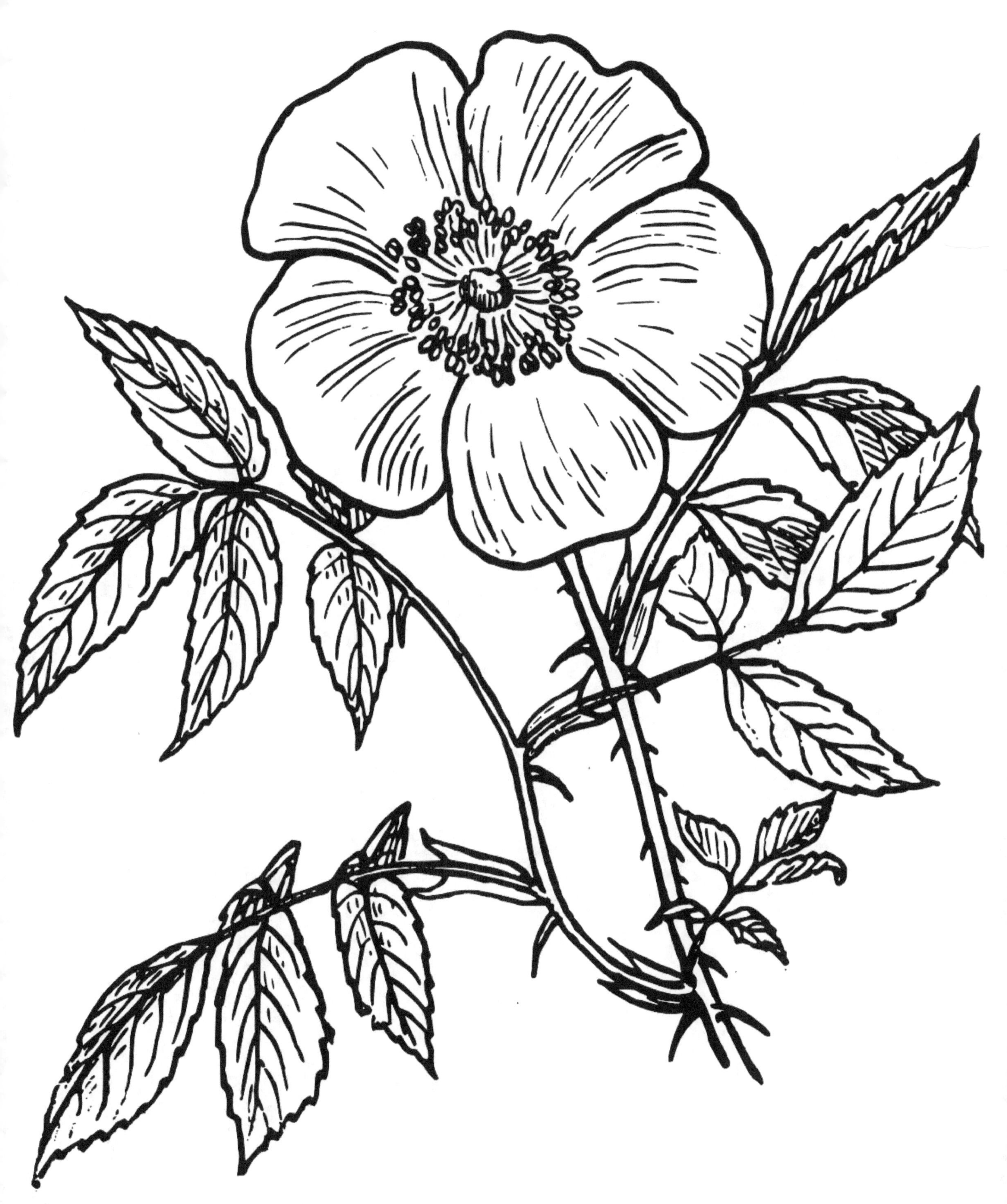

Doctor says to his patient: "Your liver results are back. And frankly, they're very surprising considering that I only allowed you one fizzy drink per week."

The old patient shrugs: "Do you really think you are the only doctor I am going to?"

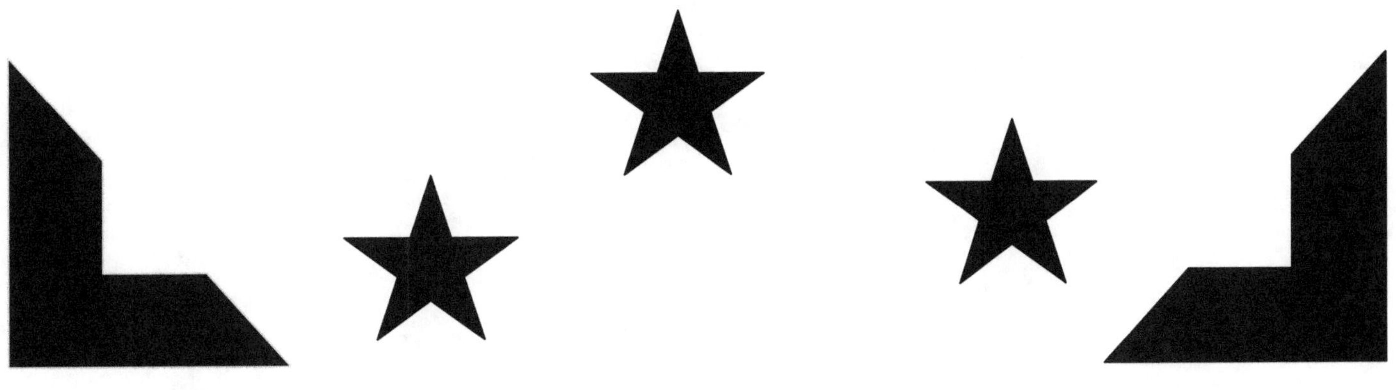

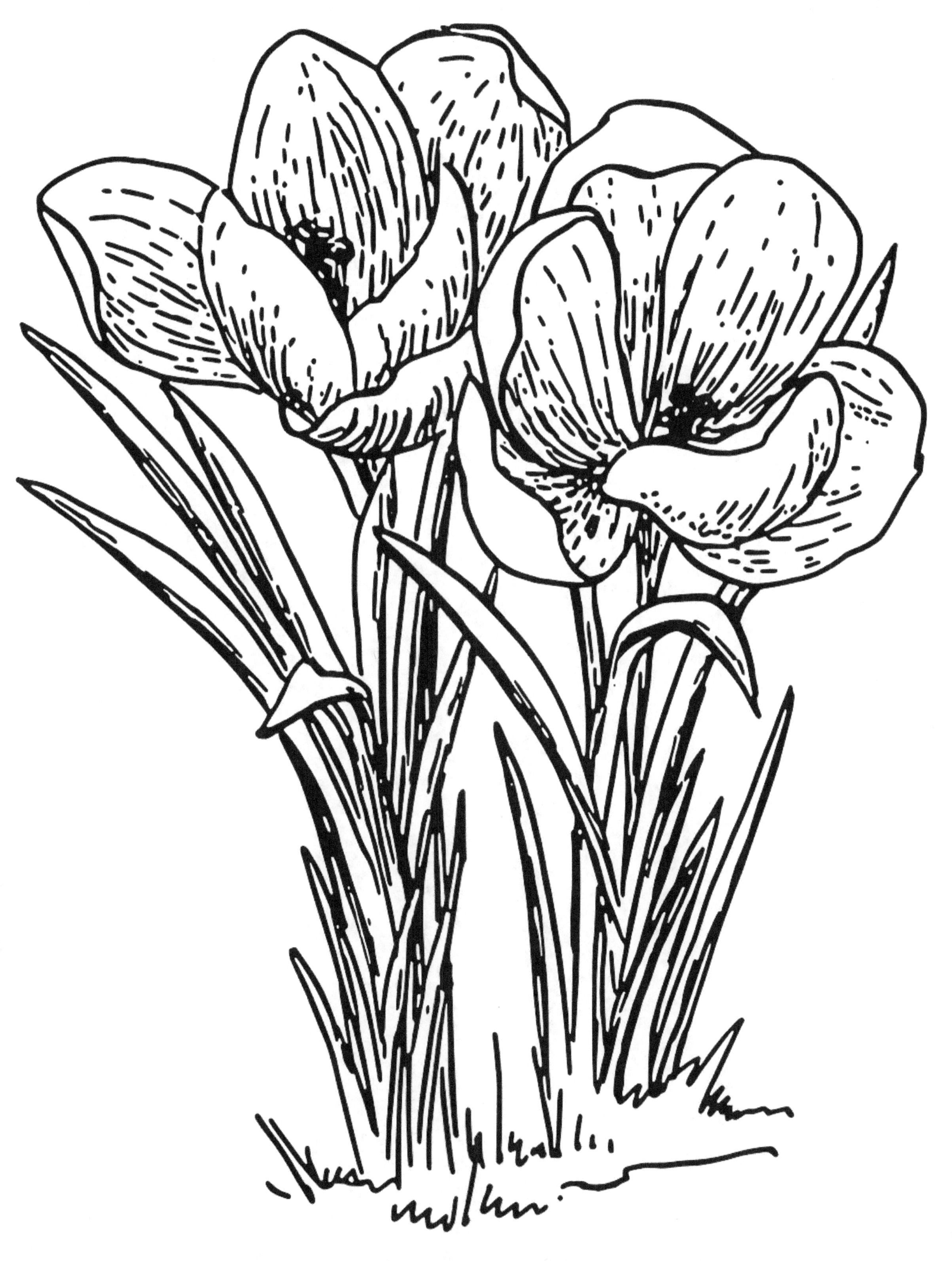

I can't believe my eyes, I just saw a grandpa with a walking stick helping a teenager who was staring into his phone to cross the road!

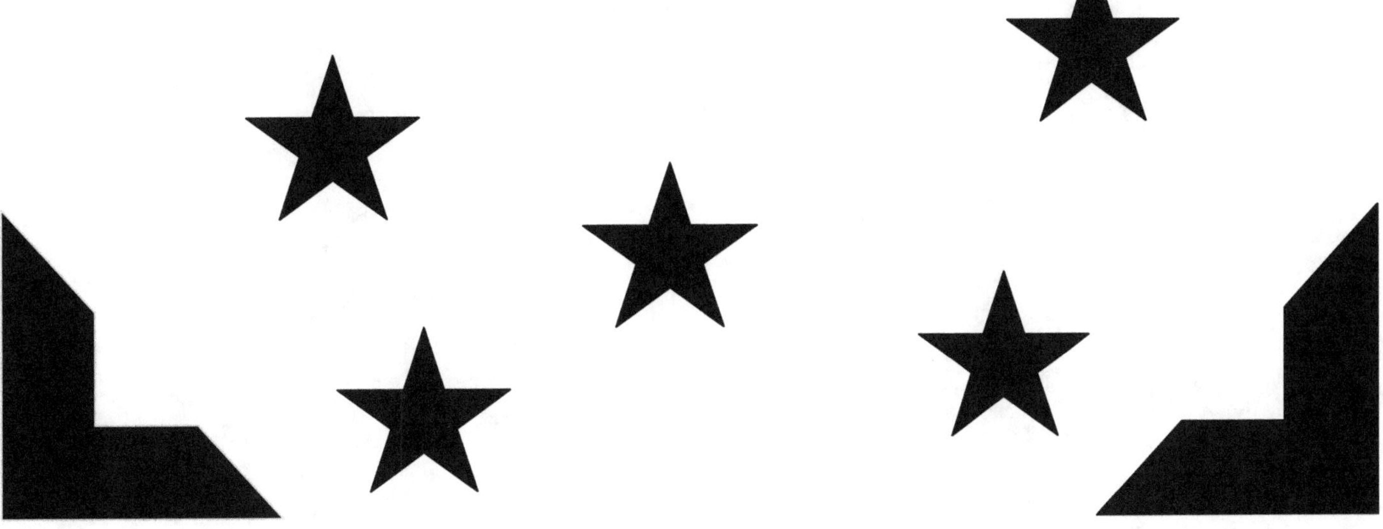

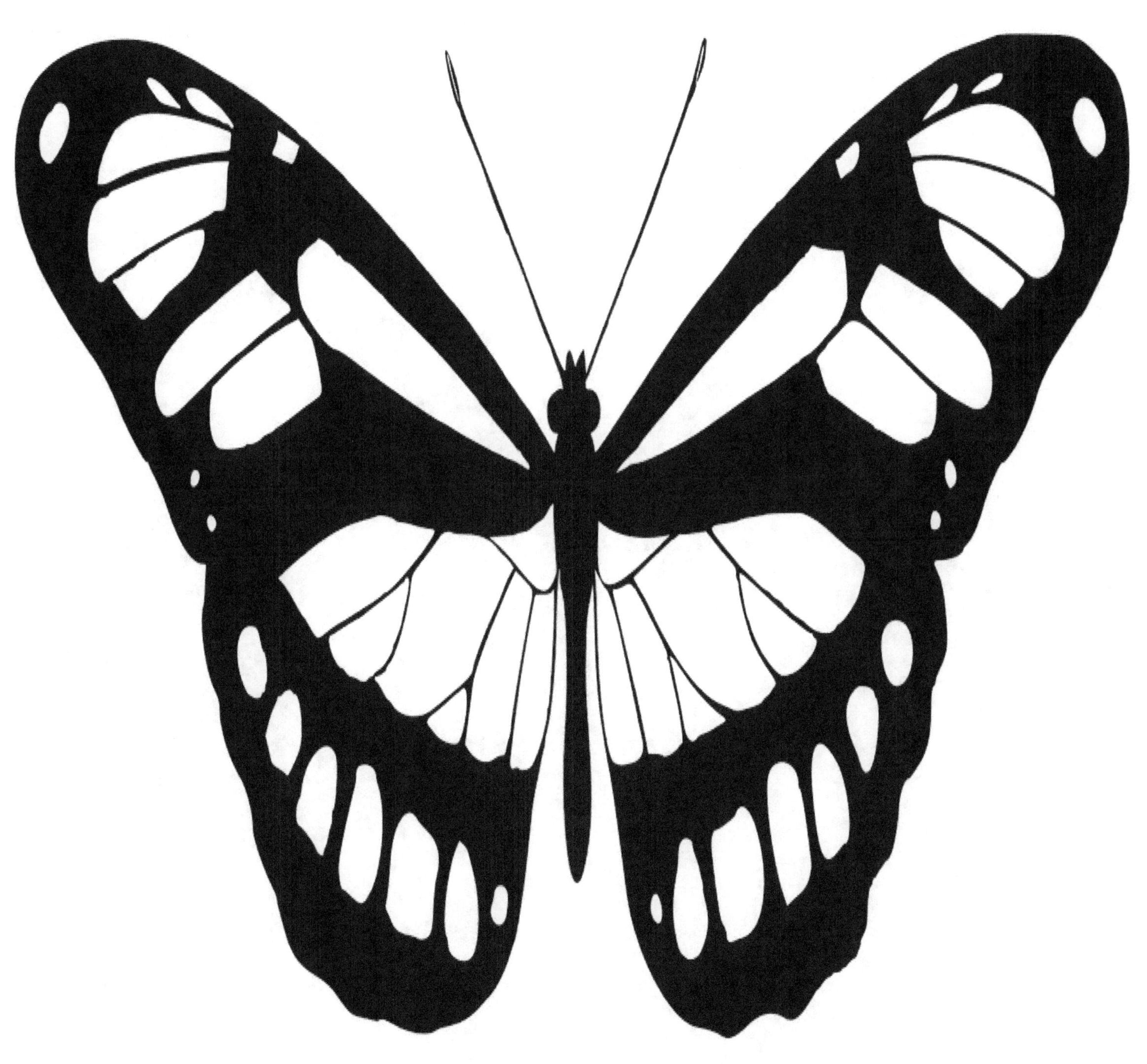

I sent my grandson a "Get better soon" card.

He's not ill or anything, but he could definitely get better.

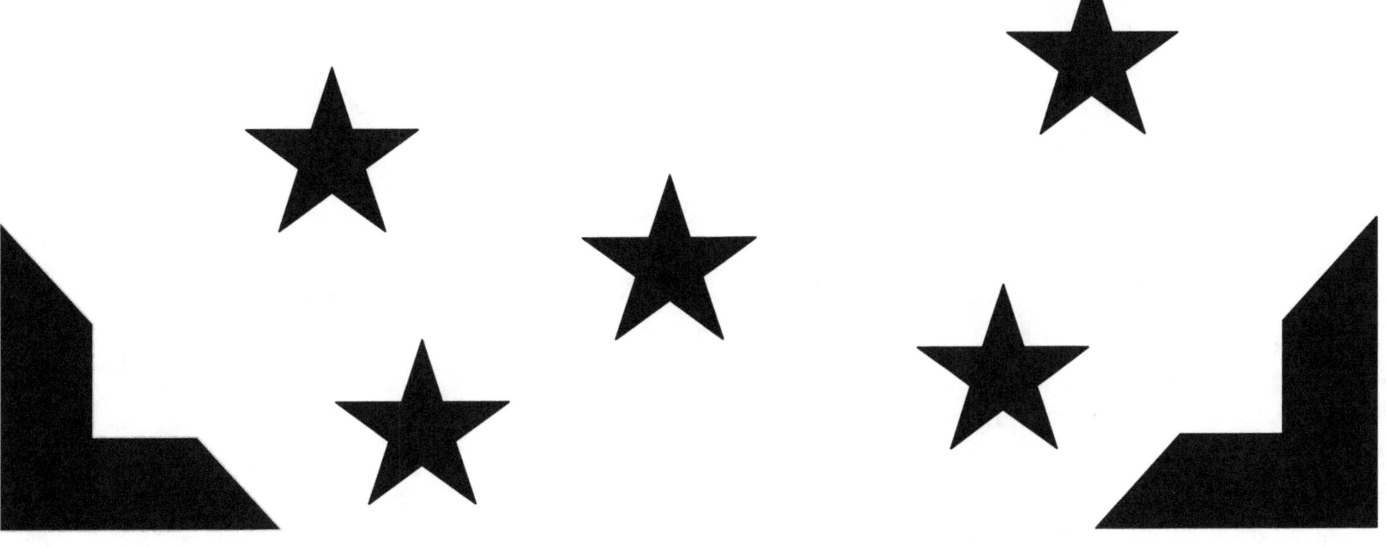

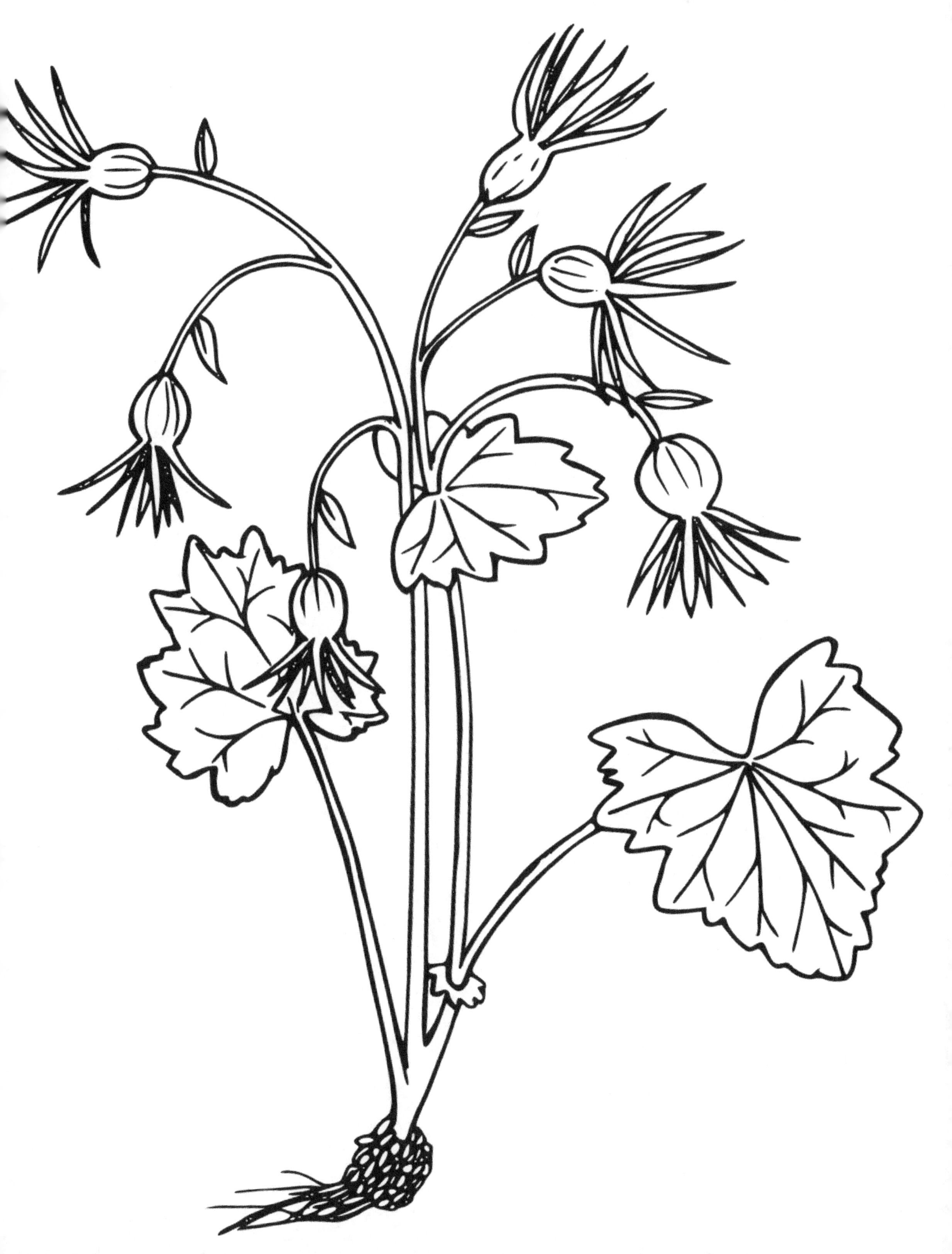

A couple with thirteen grandchildren decided to go on a date, they needed to spend quality time with just the two of them.

The man asked the waiter: "Can you bring me what the lady at the next table is having please?"

Waiter: "Sorry, Sir, but I'm pretty sure she wants to eat it herself."

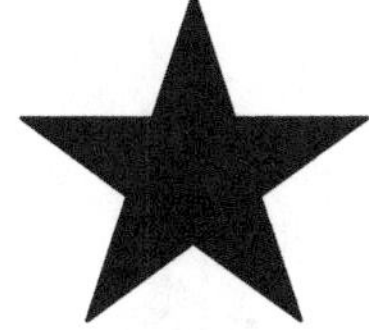

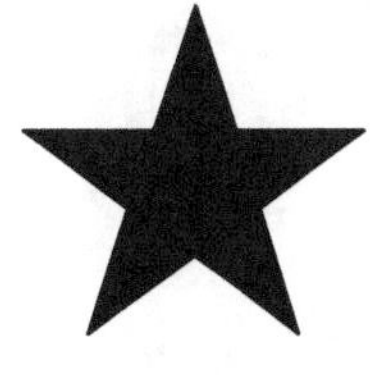

Later on they decided that they wanted to eat steak, but there was a problem.

"Waiter, the steak smells very strongly of...
I hate to say this but, it smells of urine!"
- The waiter backs up 3 steps and asks, "How's that now?

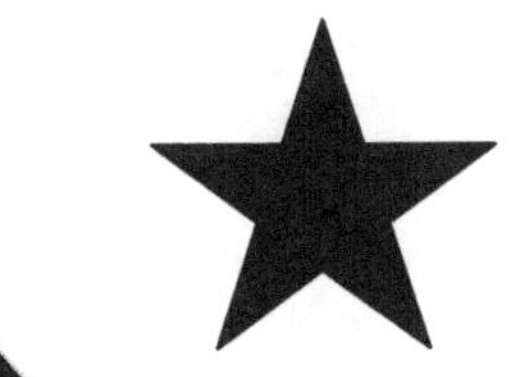
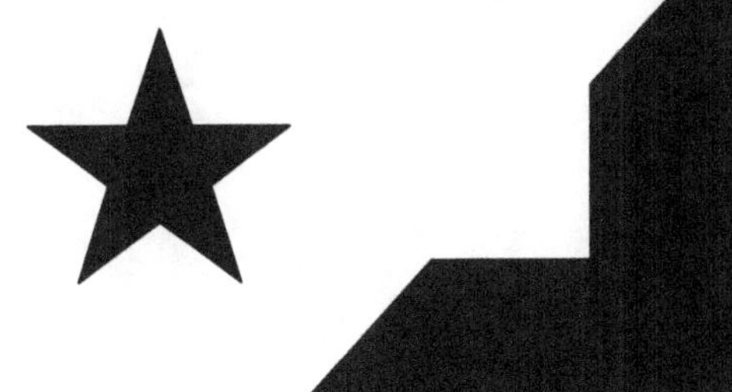

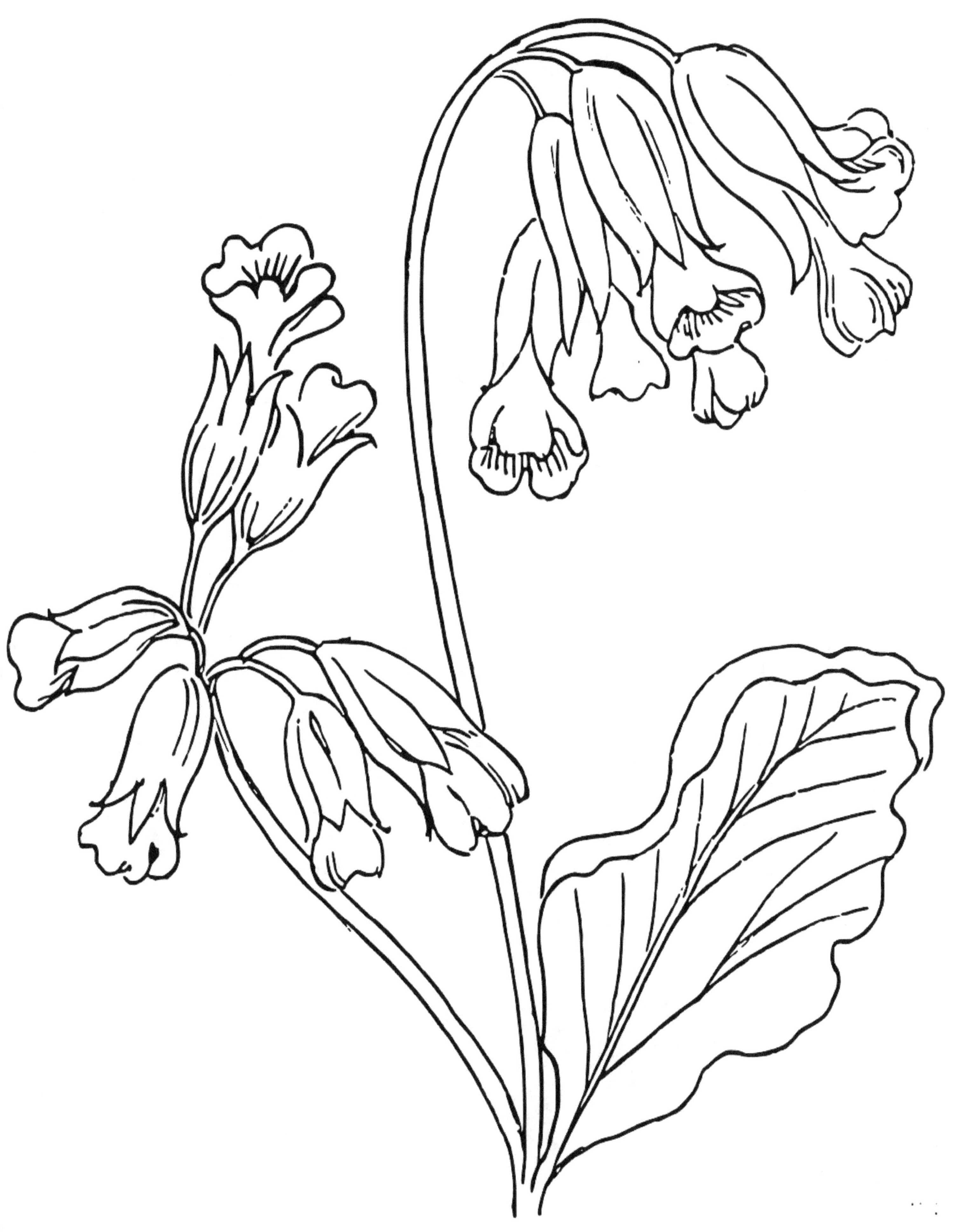

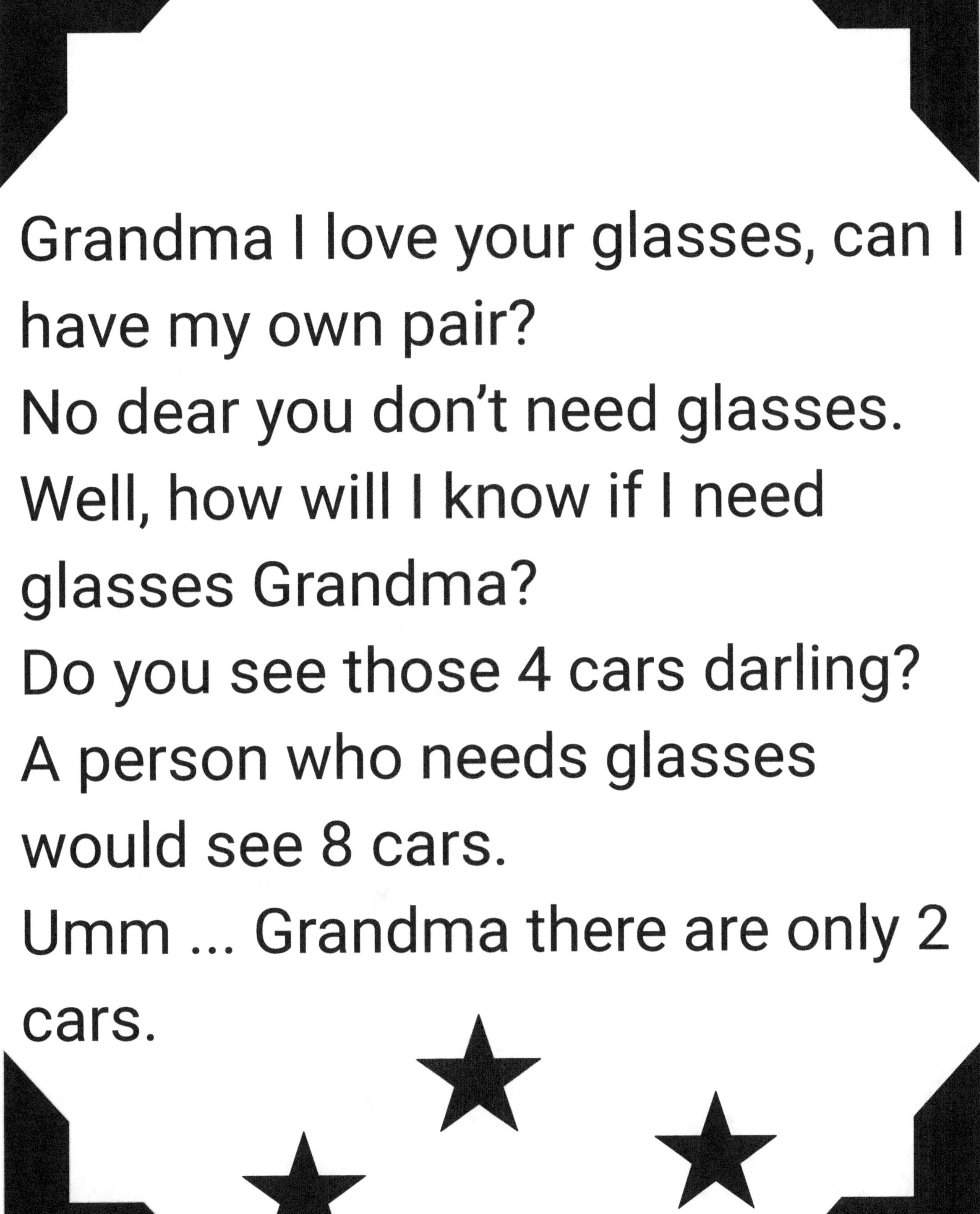

Grandma I love your glasses, can I have my own pair?

No dear you don't need glasses.

Well, how will I know if I need glasses Grandma?

Do you see those 4 cars darling?

A person who needs glasses would see 8 cars.

Umm ... Grandma there are only 2 cars.

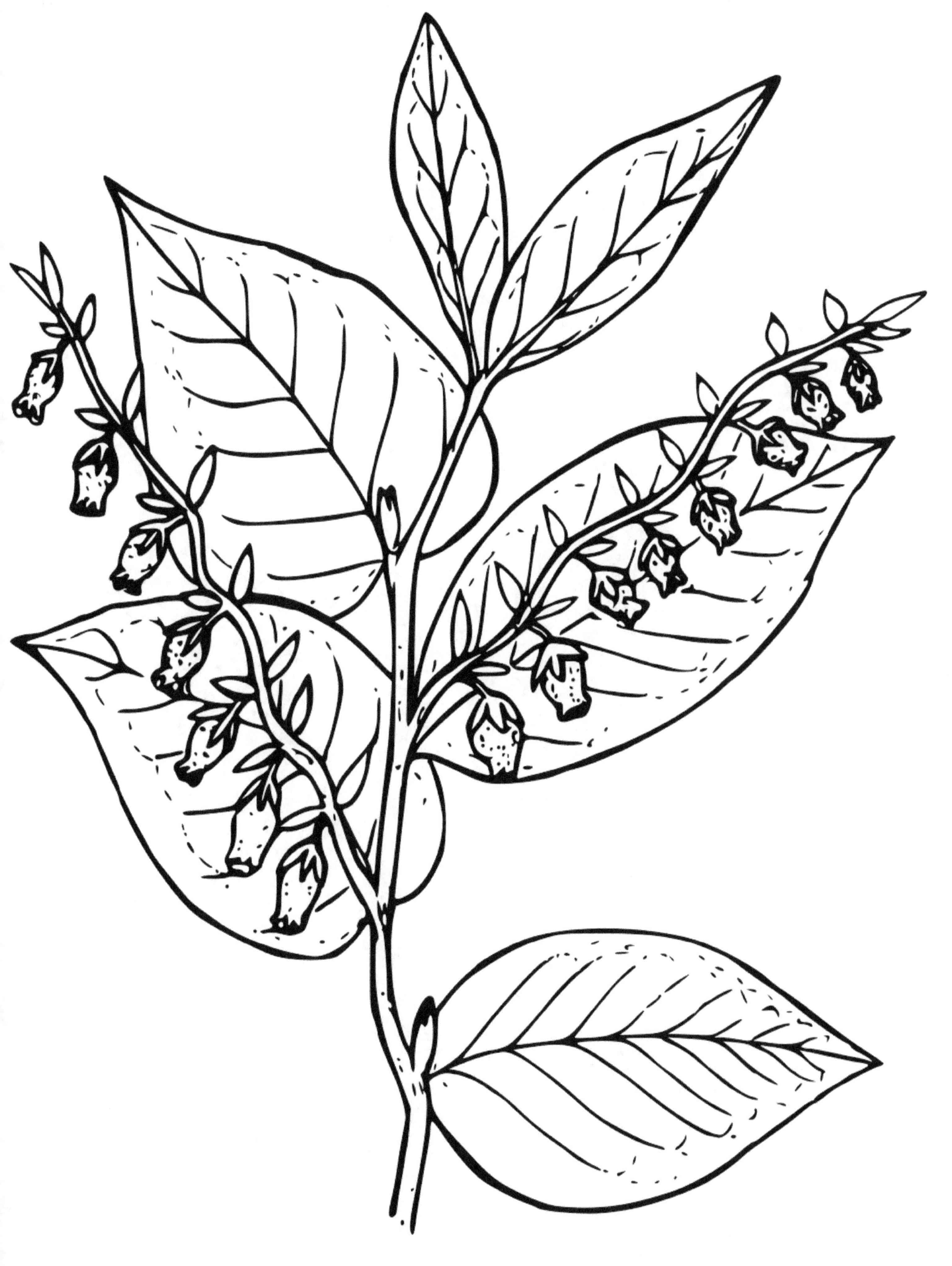

A 63 year old mother and her daughter were having tea together.

"Darling, I've been meaning to tell you that your dad has a shopping problem.

"What, so is Dad a shopaholic?"

"No I am, but he's the one who suffers."

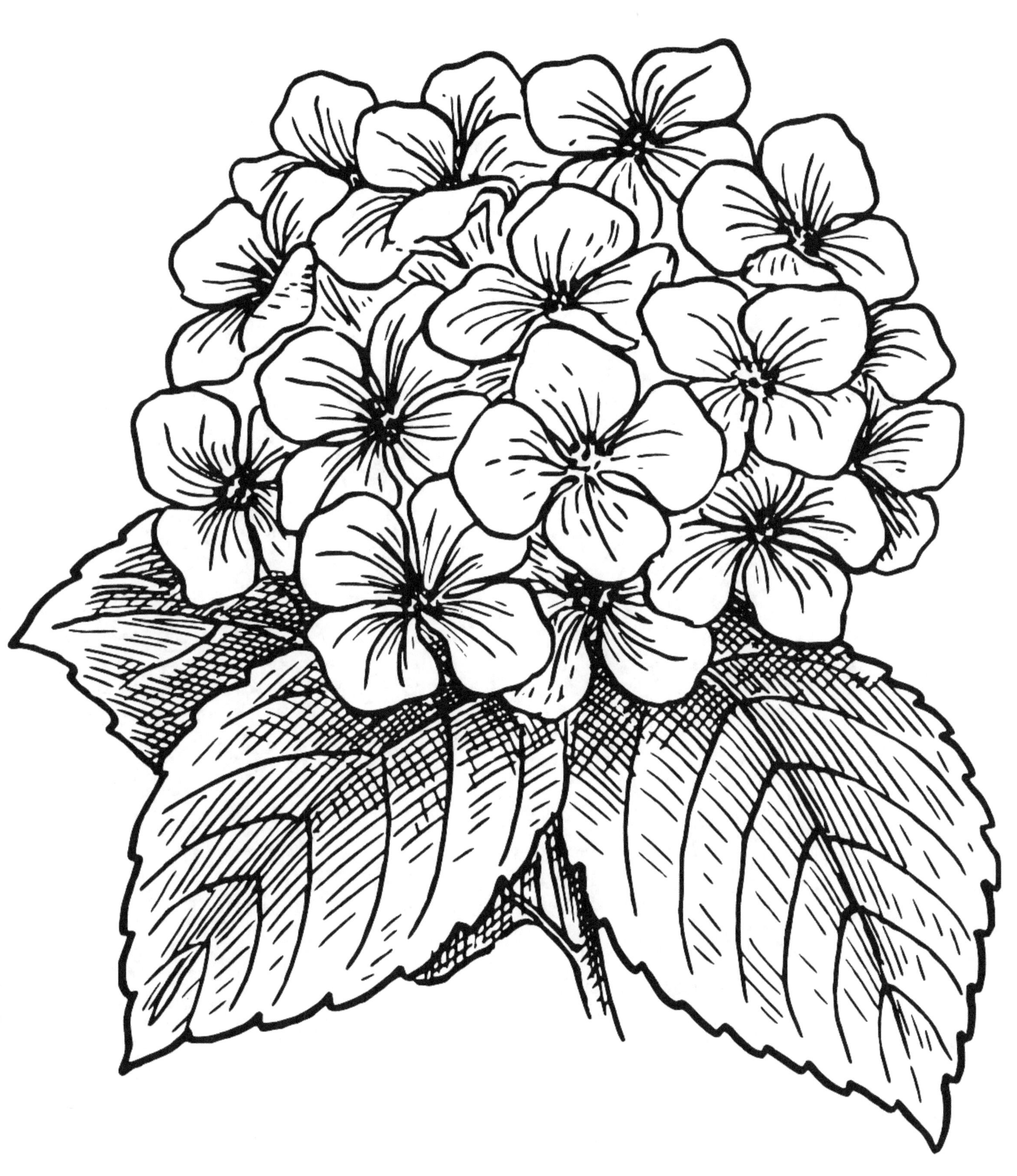

A nurse accidentally mixes up her patient's medication. Bob was given a laxative instead of cough syrup.

A few hours later Bob was missing from lunch. He was coming out of the bathroom when the nurse asked, "Are you still coughing Bob?"
Bob replies: "No. I'm afraid to."

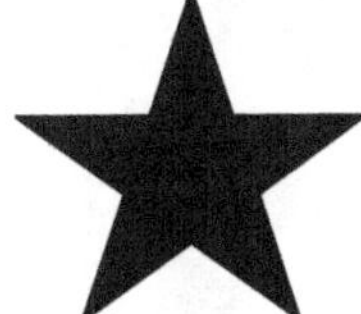

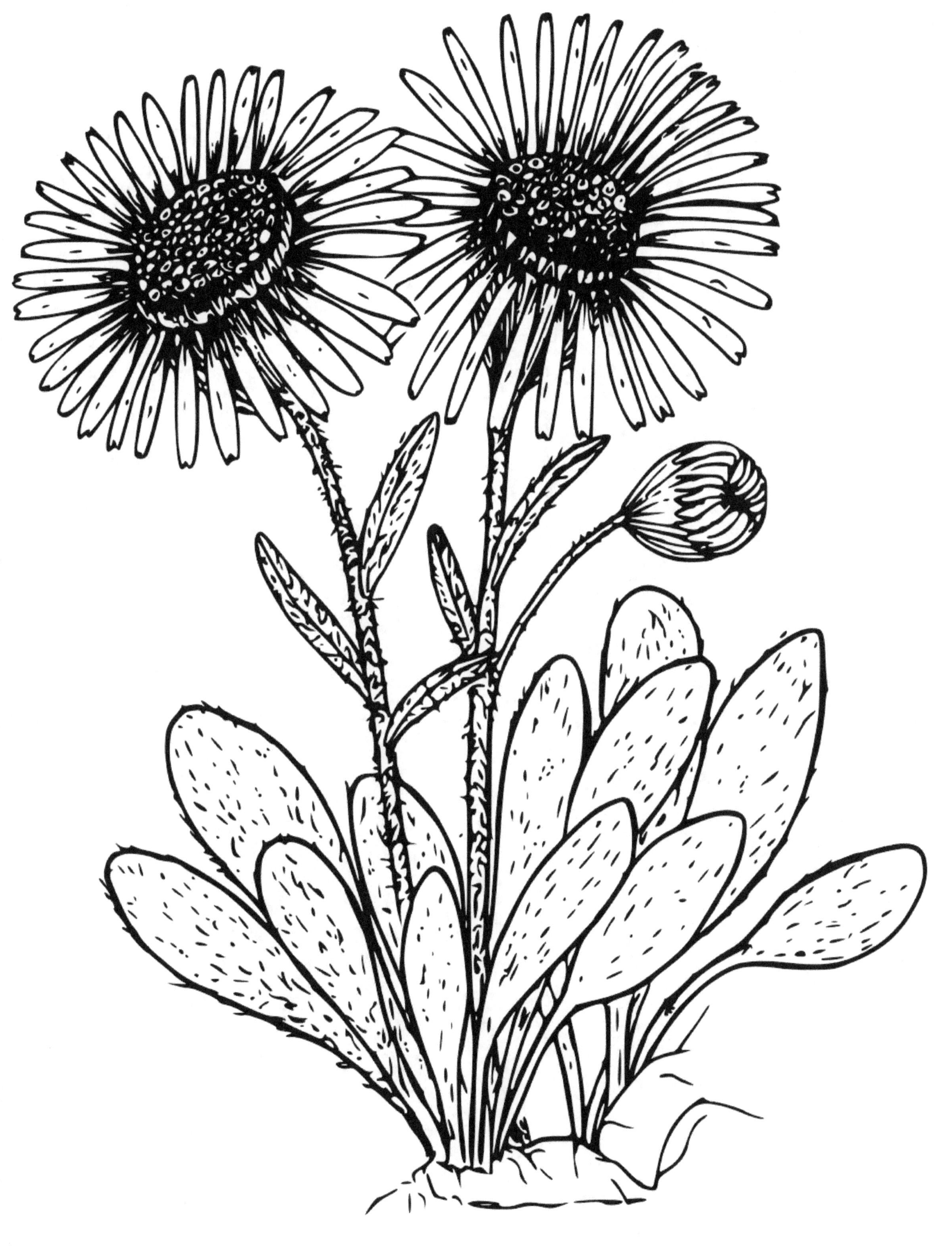

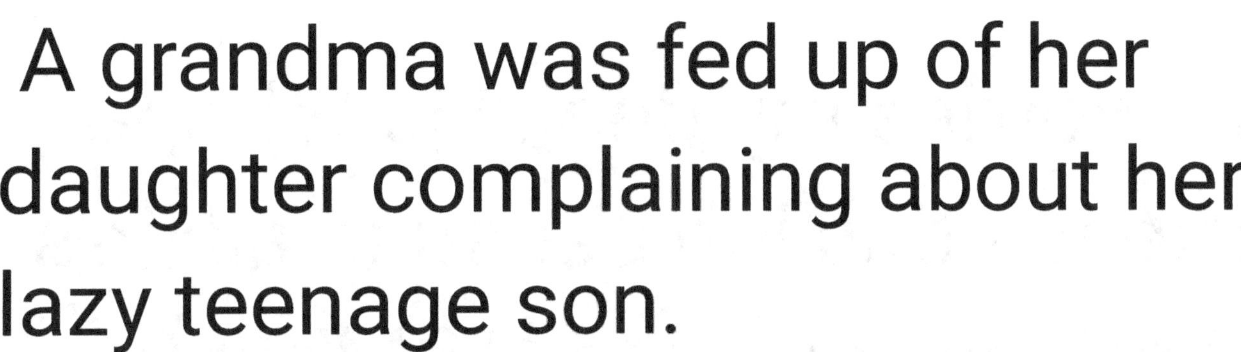

 A grandma was fed up of her daughter complaining about her lazy teenage son.

So the Grandma decided to get her Grandson a job at an M&M factory.

"It's his first day today at the M&M factory, thanks again Mum for getting my son this job.

"No worries my dear, I just hope he keeps this job because all he's got to do is sort the M&M's into bags.

Later that day the son arrived home.

"How was your day sweetie? Asked his mother.

"Erm, I was fired mum! Replied her son.

"Fired?" All you had to do was put M&M's into a bag."

That's what I thought! But I didn't see "M's" so I kept throwing out all the "W's".

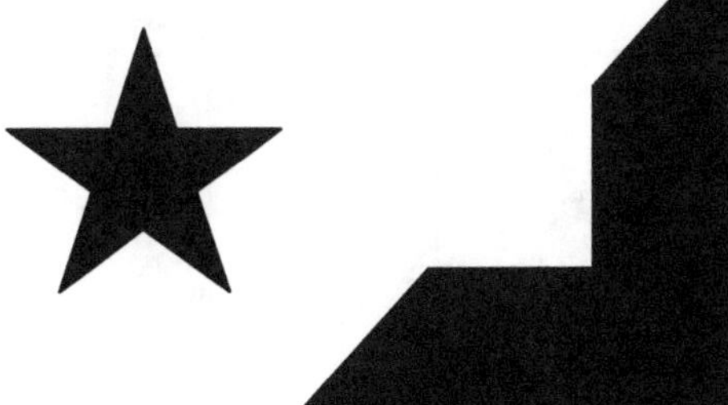

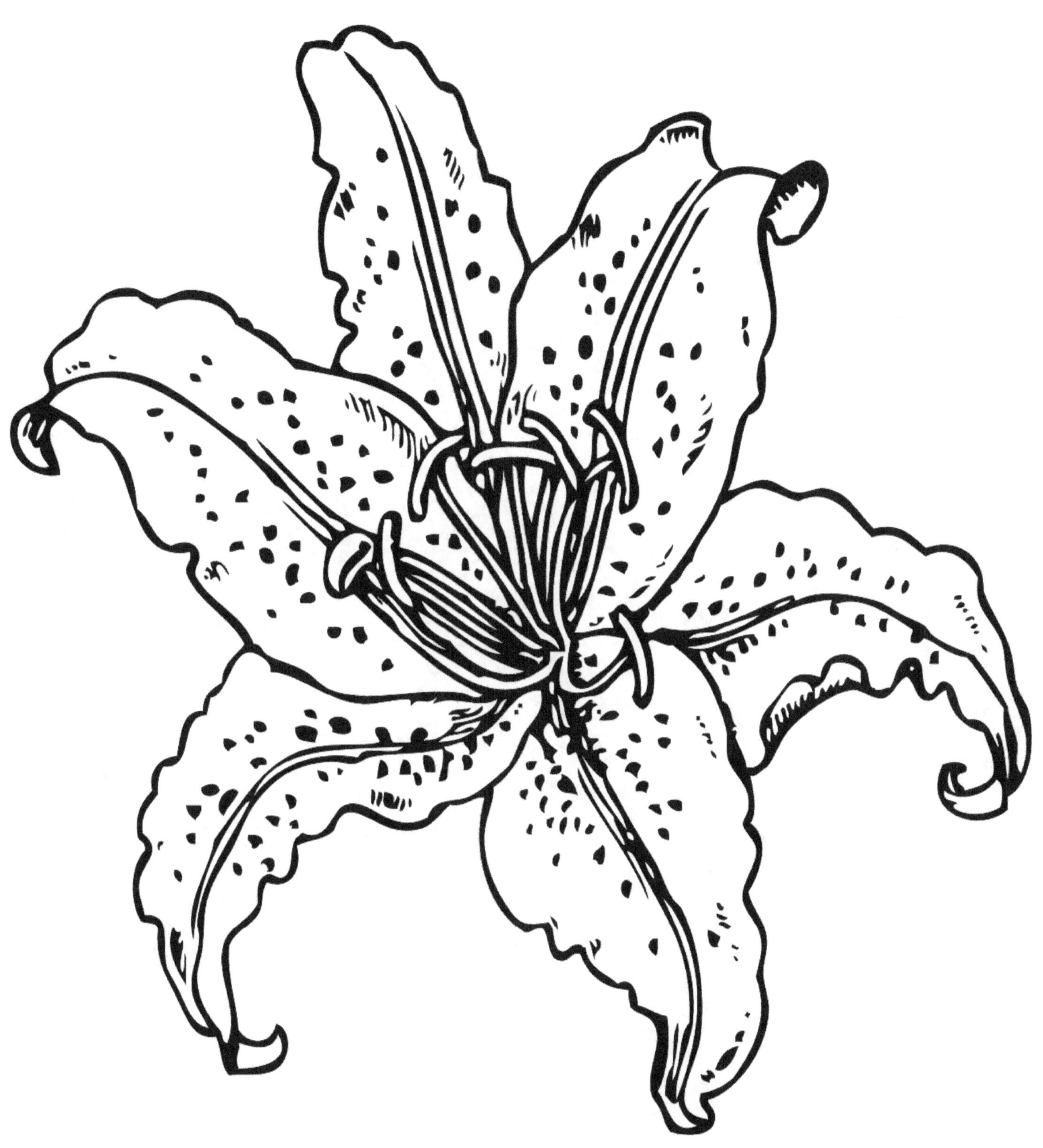

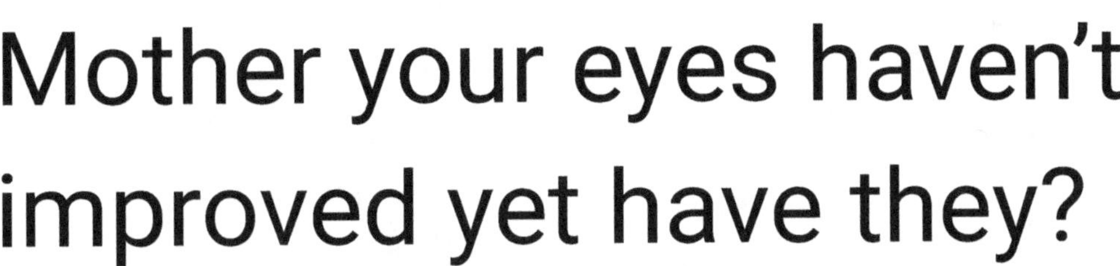

Mother your eyes haven't
improved yet have they?

What do you mean?

You came all the way from your
house using your step ladder
instead of your walking frame!

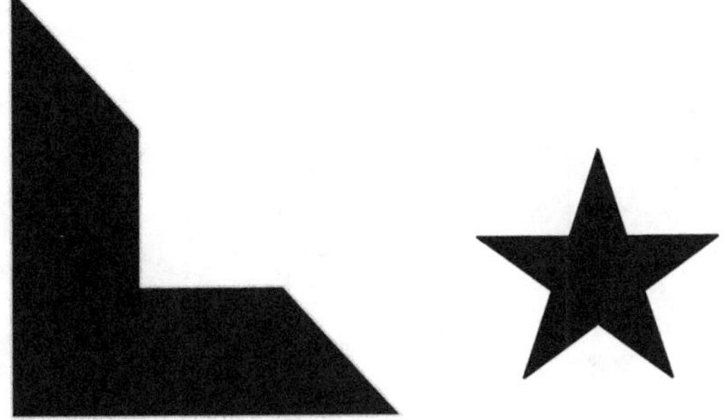

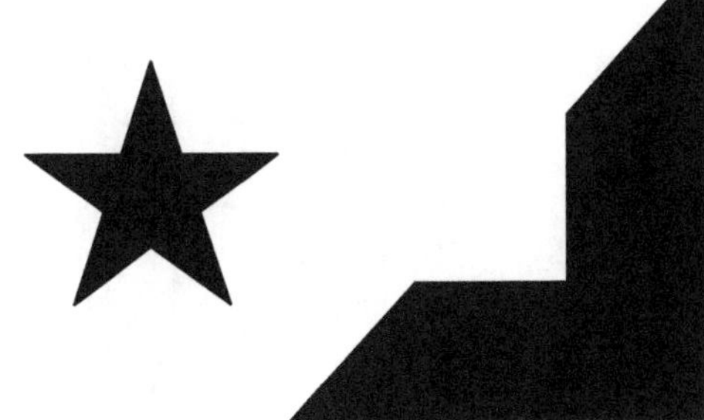

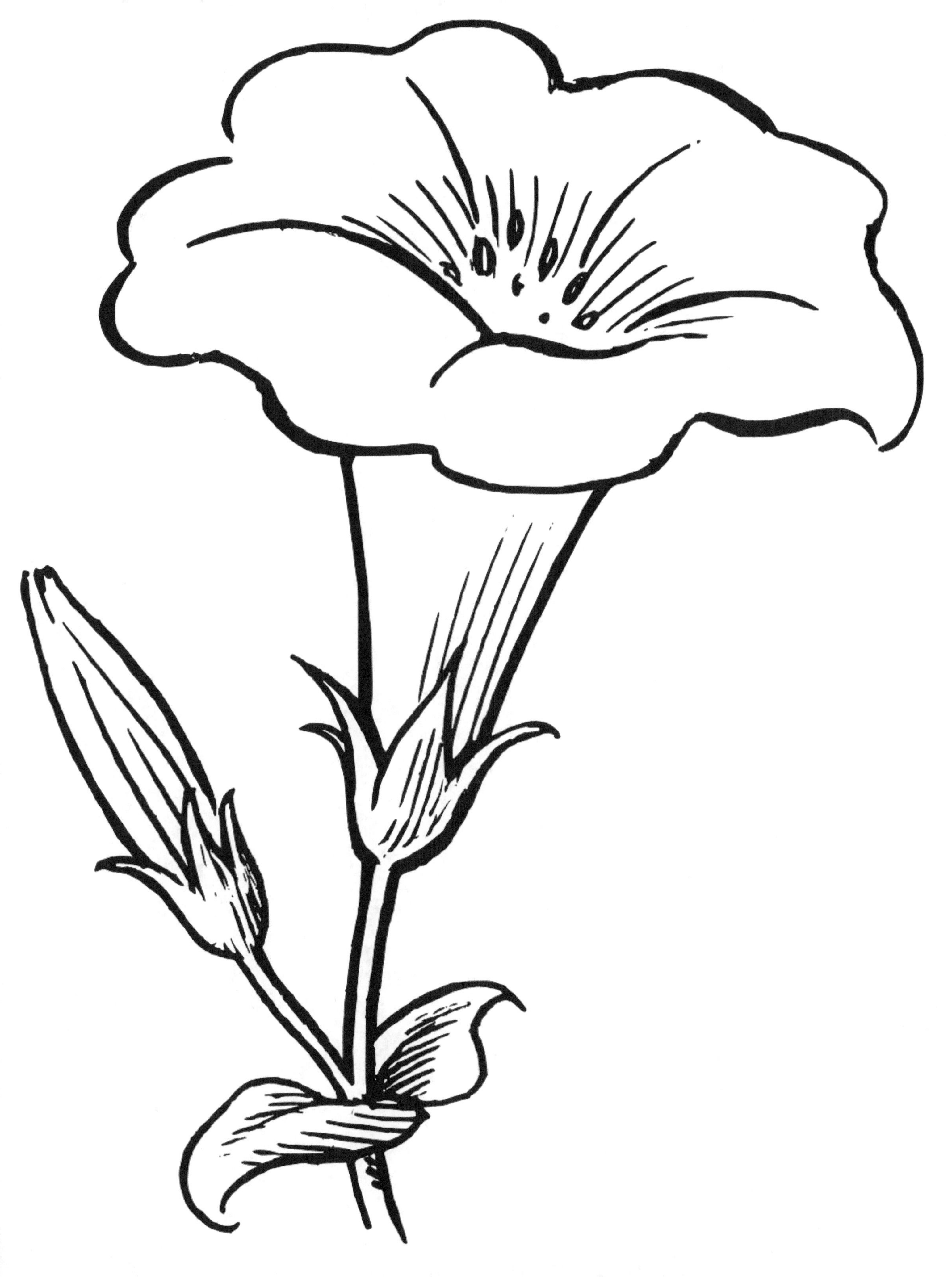

Betty's grandad lived on a farm.
On Betty's first day on the farm she gave the cow a huge stack of hay.

On Betty's second day on the farm she gave the cow a pile of grass.

On Betty's third day she gave the cow 15 pieces of corn.
On each day Betty's Grandad saw what Betty was doing and shook his head.

On the fourth day he said, "Don't pamper the cow love, you'll get spoiled milk."

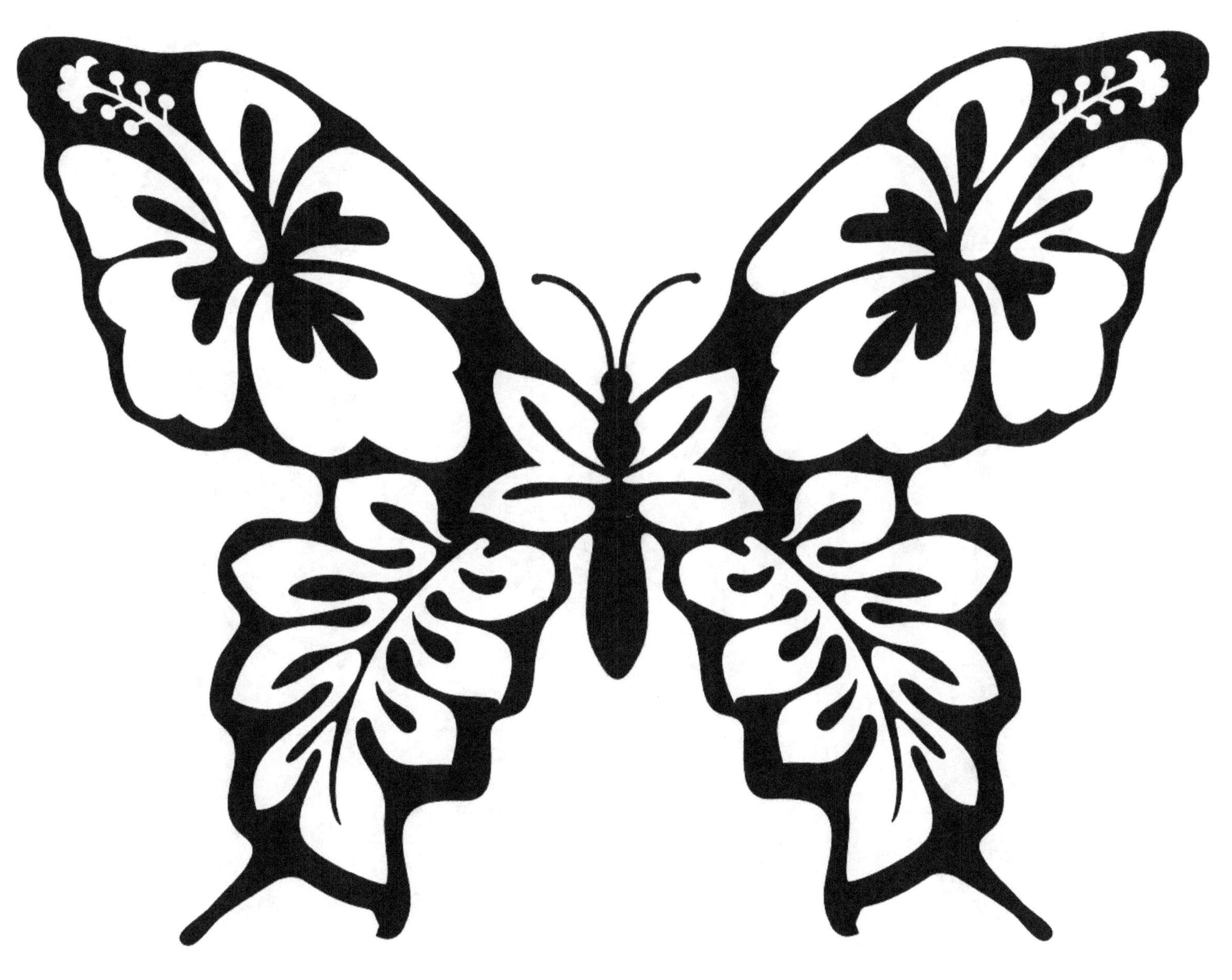

An older woman points to another older couple across the road to her husband: "Just look at that couple, they are so in love. He is holding her hand, he kissed her and he held the door open for her, why can't you do the same?"

"I'm so disgusted! I don't even know her."

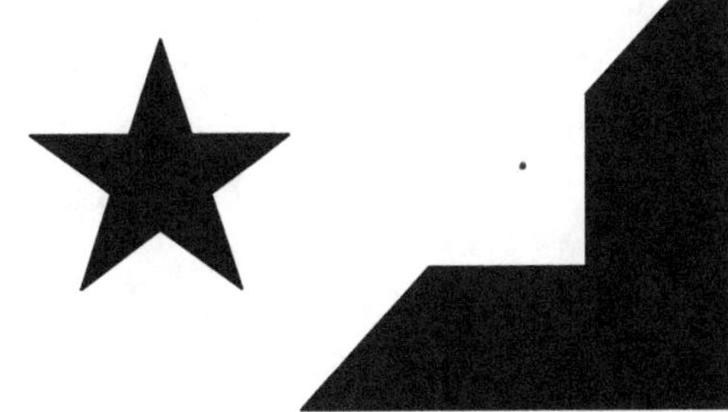

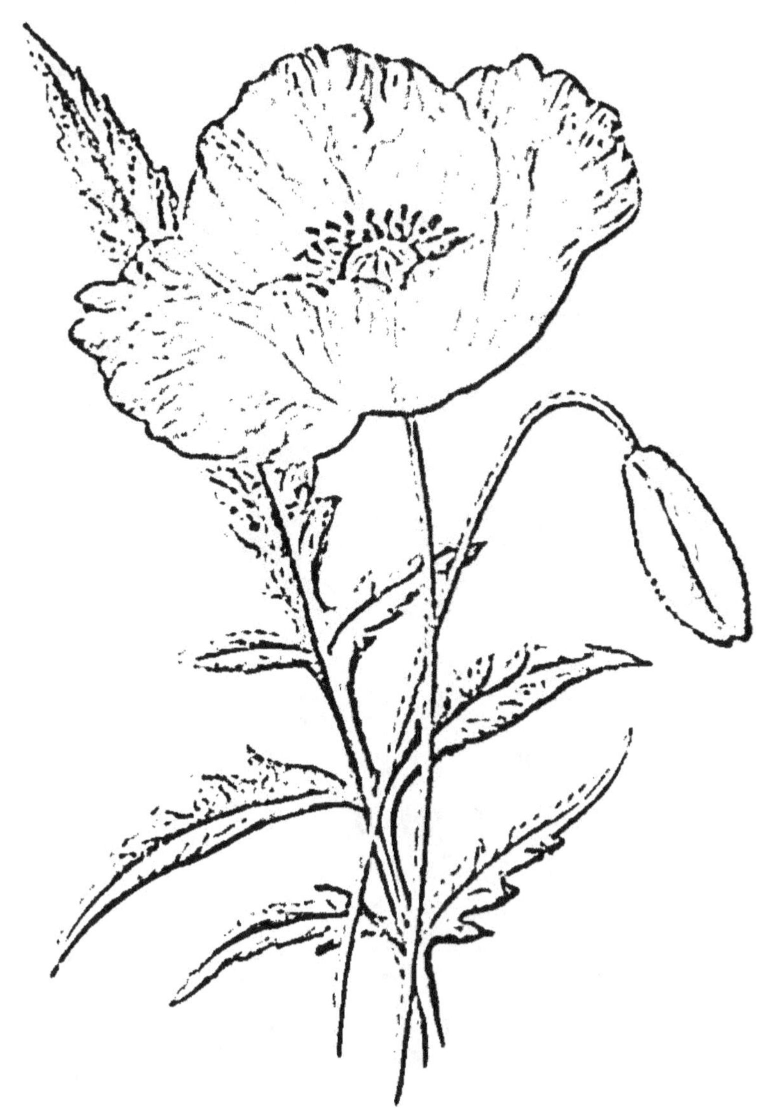

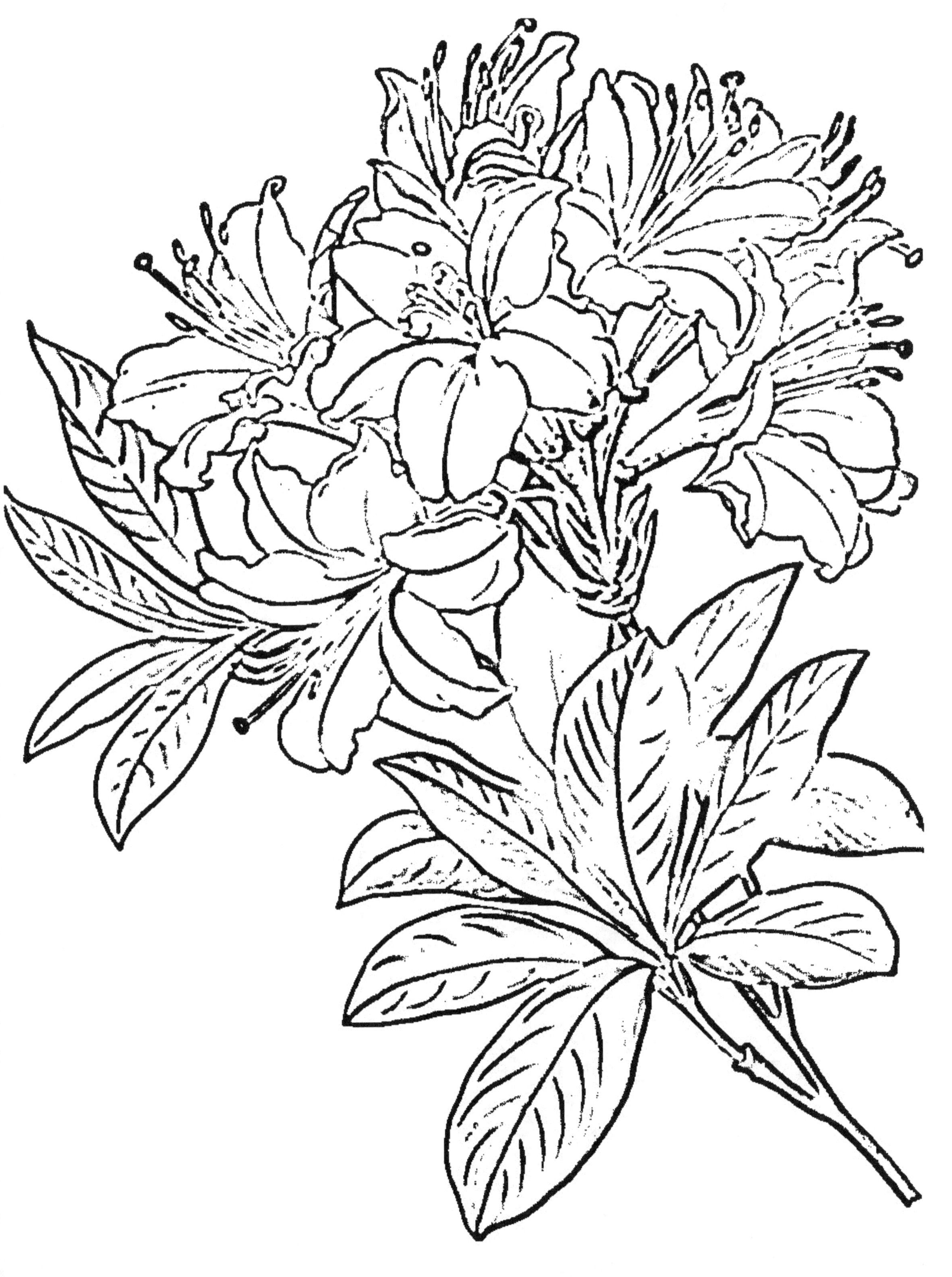

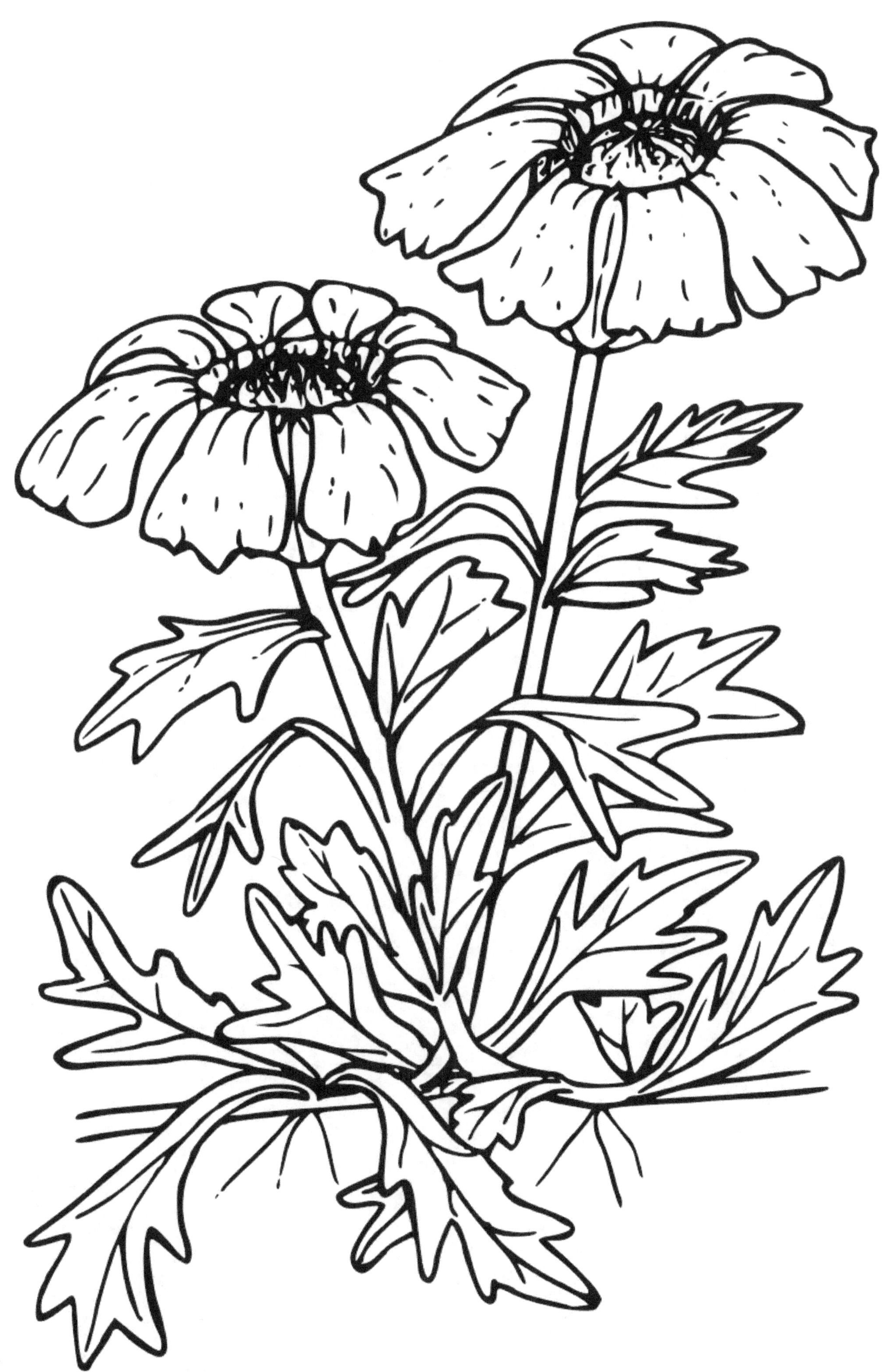

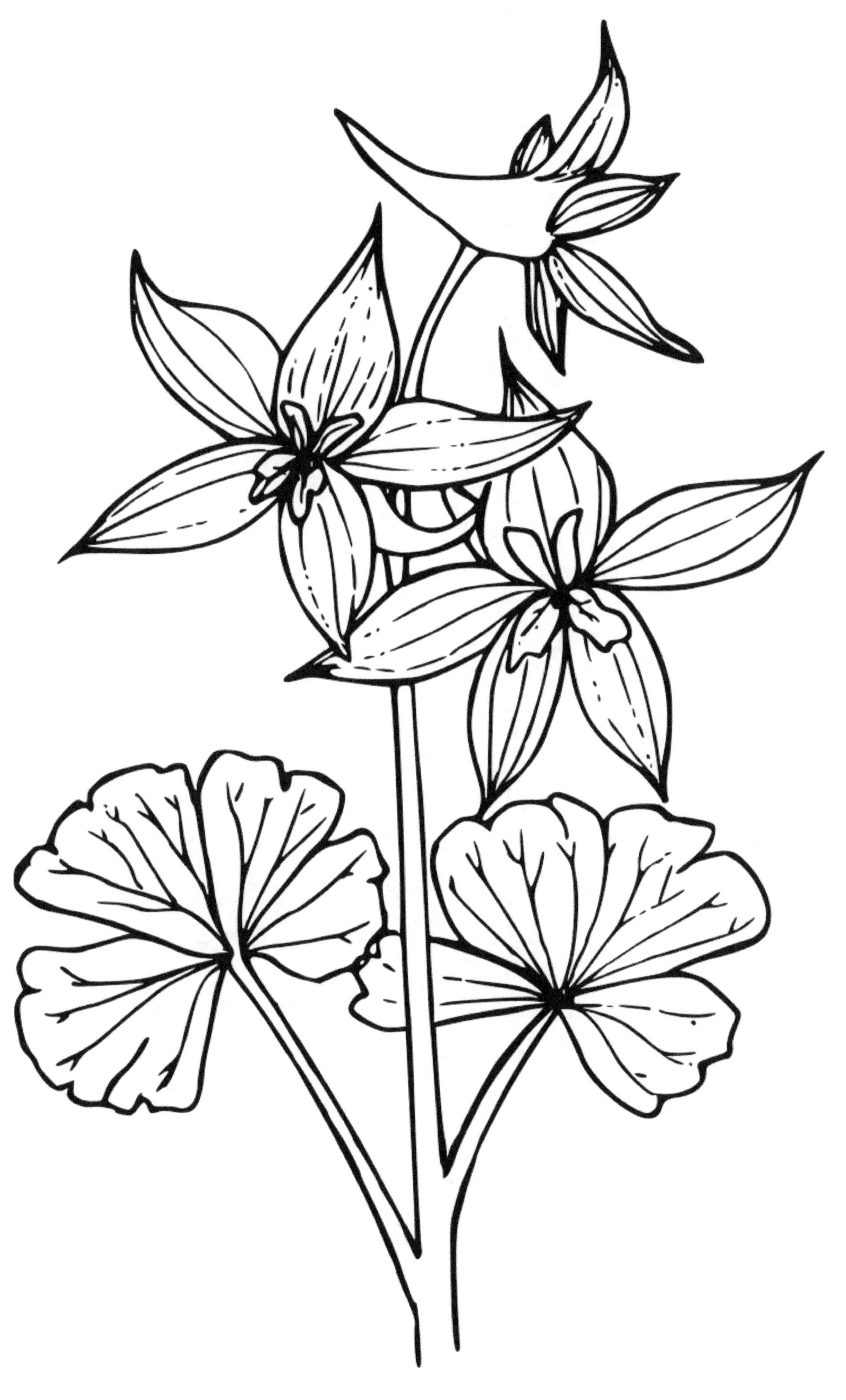

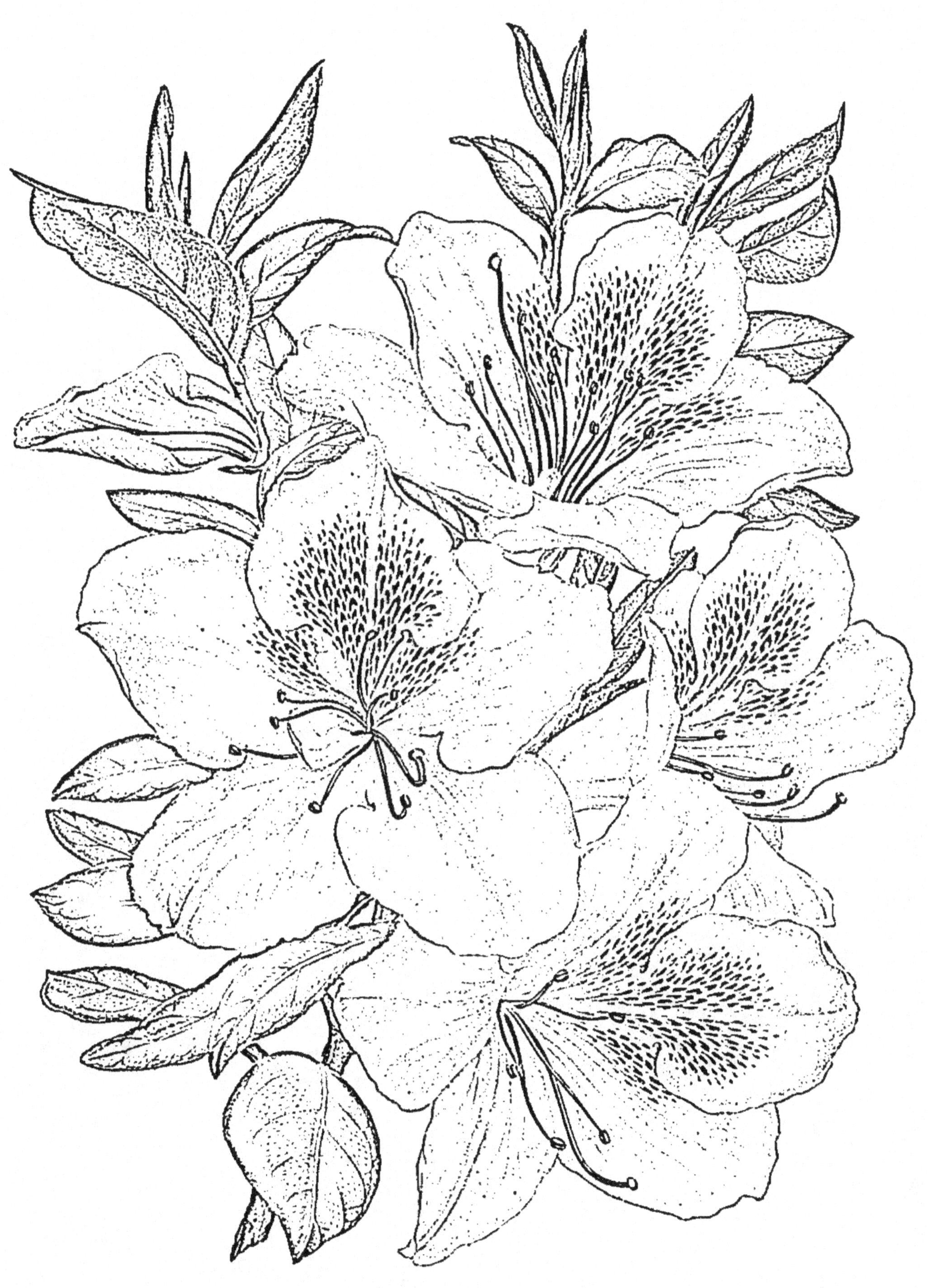

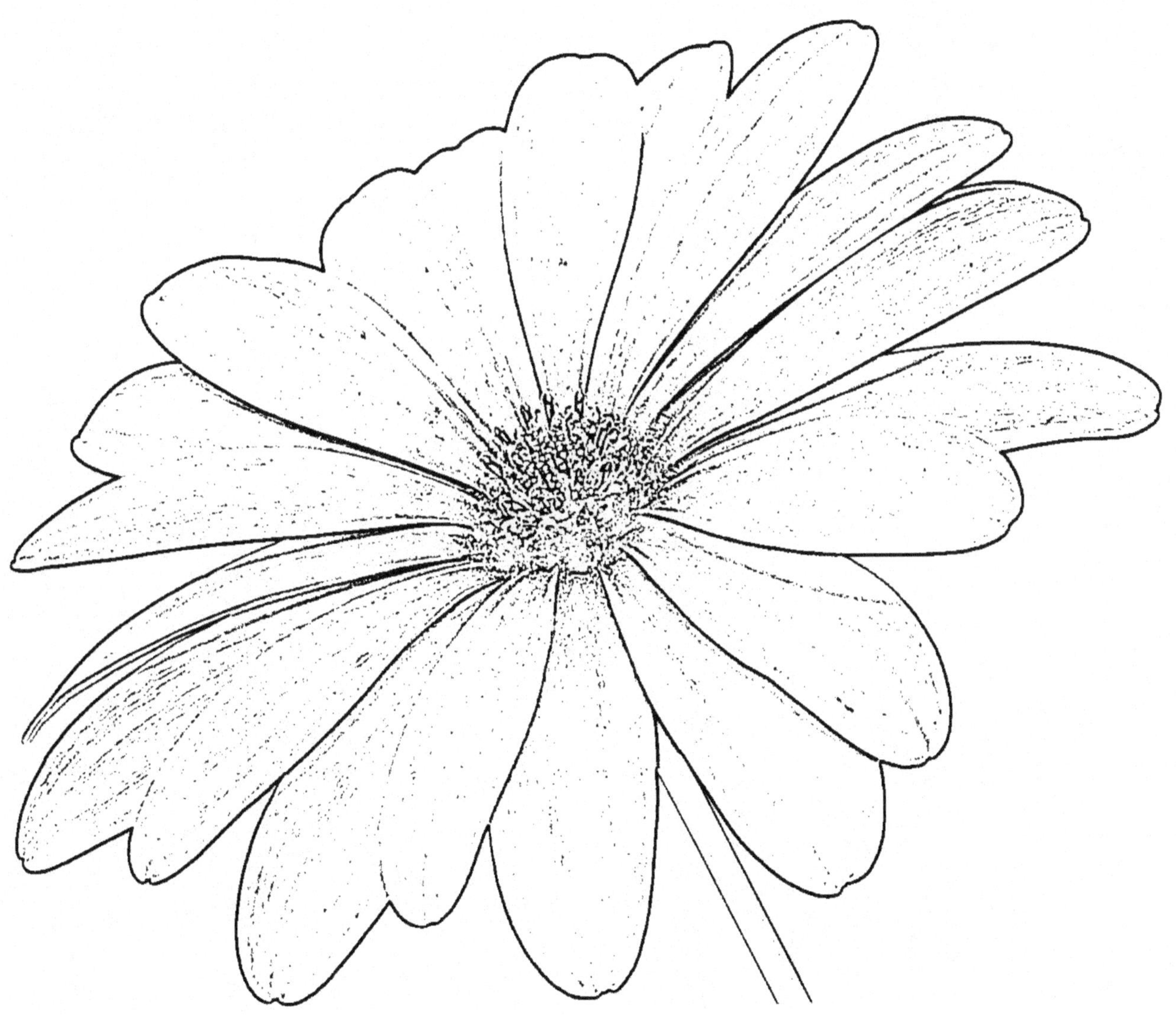

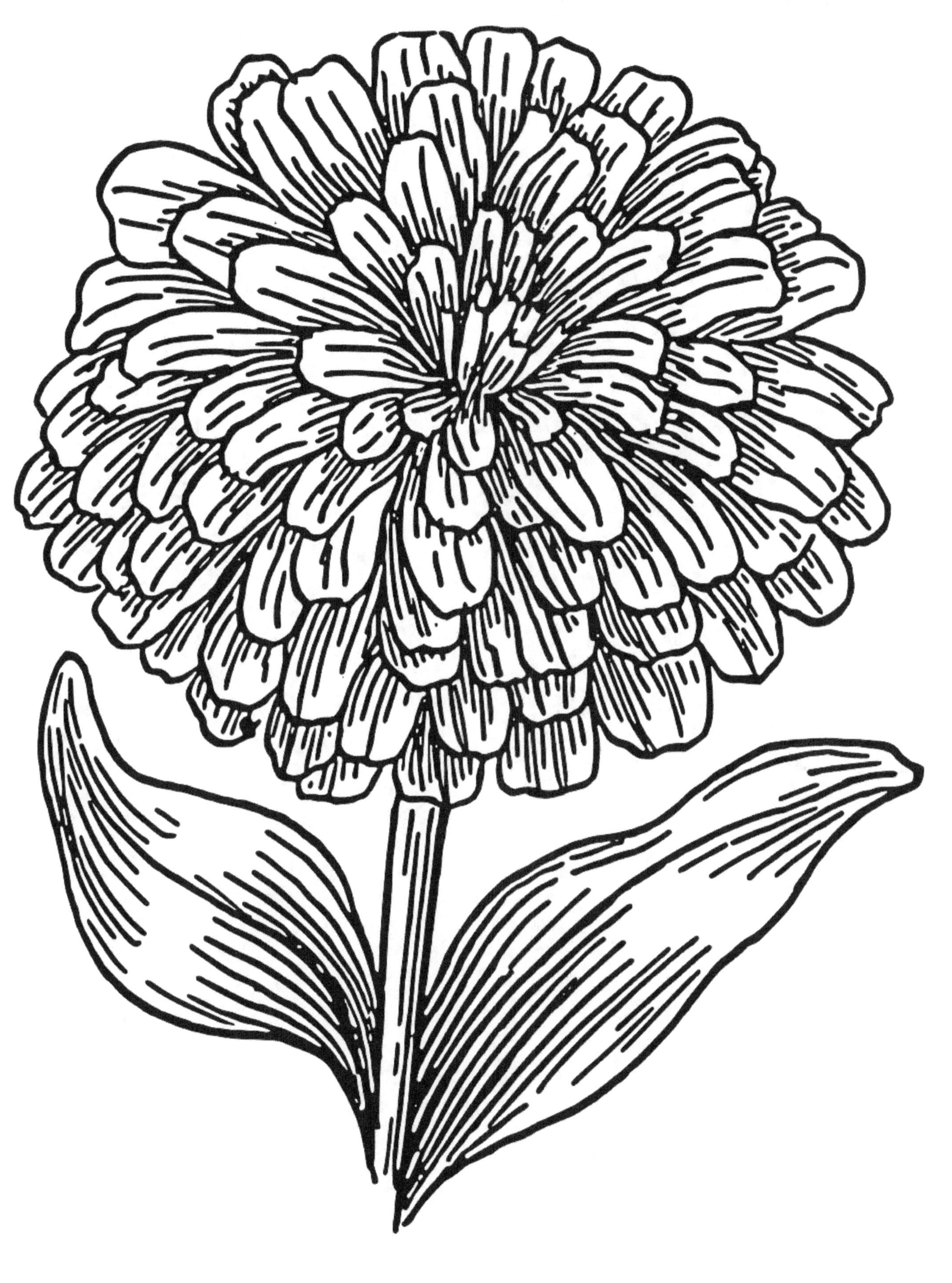

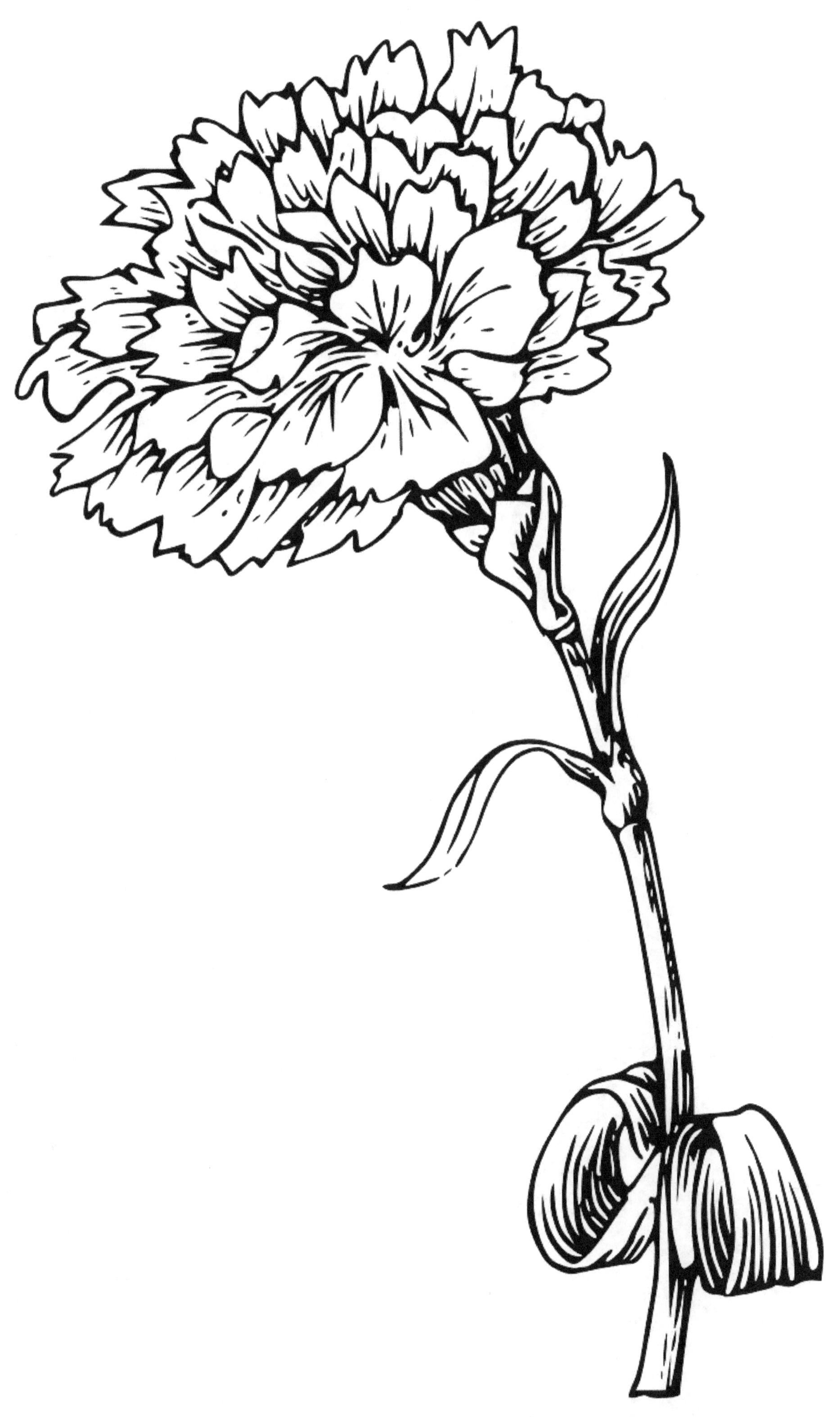

We hoped you enjoyed this
book.

Please remember to write a
review.

Keep Smiling!

www.ingramcontent.com/pod-product-compliance
Lightning Source LLC
Chambersburg PA
CBHW081314250726
48662CB00008B/2565